NUTRITION AND DIET RESEARCH PROGRESS

PARENTERAL NUTRITION

POLICIES AND PROCEDURES, SAFE PRACTICES AND POTENTIAL COMPLICATIONS

NUTRITION AND DIET RESEARCH PROGRESS

Additional books in this series can be found on Nova's website under the Series tab.

Additional e-books in this series can be found on Nova's website under the e-book tab.

NUTRITION AND DIET RESEARCH PROGRESS

PARENTERAL NUTRITION

POLICIES AND PROCEDURES, SAFE PRACTICES AND POTENTIAL COMPLICATIONS

SHANA LELIO
EDITOR

New York

For permission to use material from this book please contact us:
Telephone 631-231-7269; Fax 631-231-8175
Web Site: http://www.novapublishers.com

Additional color graphics may be available in the e-book version of this book.

Library of Congress Cataloging-in-Publication Data

ISBN: 978-1-63321-112-4

Library of Congress Control Number: 2014940582

Published by Nova Science Publishers, Inc. † New York

Contents

Preface

Parenteral nutrition (PN) is the feeding modality of choice for patients with non-functional gastrointestinal (GI) tracts who are unable to maintain their nutrition and hydration enterally. Parenteral nutrition is a complex therapy involving the intravenous infusion of macro and micronutrients directly into the bloodstream for optimal absorption. The main components of parenteral formulas include dextrose, amino acids and lipids. Although PN is a lifesaving therapy for many patients, it is associated with serious short and long-term complications that can be life-threatening. Therefore, selection of the appropriate patient for parenteral therapy is crucial. This book discusses the policies, procedures, safe practices and potential of parenteral nutrition, as well as nutritional considerations for head and neck cancer patients; nutrition support teams and the role of registered dieticians; parenteral nutrition associated liver disease; and refeeding syndrome in children.

Chapter 1 – Parenteral nutrition (PN) is the feeding modality of choice for patients with non-functional gastrointestinal (GI) tracts who are unable to maintain their nutrition and hydration enterally. Although it is a lifesaving therapy, it is associated with serious complications. A specialized nutrition support team can help select patients who are appropriate for parenteral nutrition. There are short term and long term indications for TPN. Short-term indications include ileus, tube feeding intolerance, small bowel obstruction, bowel rest and perioperative. Long-term indications include short bowel syndrome, recurrent small bowel obstructions, intestinal fistulae, gastrointestinal dysmotility, mesenteric ischemia, inflammatory bowel disease and radiation enteritis.

Once the patient is selected and a medical plan is made, appropriate intravenous access should be placed. For those requiring short-term parenteral nutrition, peripheral intravenous access is reasonable, however it is preferred to administer parenteral nutrition through a central vein. Central venous access can be gained via peripherally inserted central catheter, central venous catheter, tunneled catheter or med port. Short-term complications of parenteral nutrition include catheter related infections, catheter related thrombosis and deep vein thrombosis, abnormal blood sugars and electrolytes, fluid overload or dehydration. Long-term complications include parenteral nutrition induced liver disease, metabolic bone disease, catheter related infections and sepsis, mechanical complications of central catheters, and catheter thrombosis and blood clots. These complications can be minimized and sometimes prevented if managed by a specialized nutrition support team or a team with good knowledge about parenteral nutrition both in the inpatient and outpatient settings.

Chapter 2 – Approximately 35-60% of all head and neck cancer patients are malnourished at the time of their diagnosis, either due to tumor burden and obstruction of intake and/or the anorexia/cachexia associated with their cancer. Most of those patients will require parentral nutrition before and after surgical treatment, adjuvant chemotherapy, and/ or radiotherapy. Moreover, head and neck cancer generally affect older population with multiple medical comorbidities that may complicate managing their nutritional needs. Nutritional interventions should be initiated before the cancer treatment begins and these interventions need to be ongoing following completion of treatment to ensure optimal outcomes for patients. A nutritional assessment must be part of all comprehensive treatment plans for patients with head and neck cancer. Alternative nutritional interventions such as immune-enhancing nutrients or anti-cytokine pharmaceutical agents may also be effective as adjuvant therapies, but more research is needed to quantify their clinical effect. This chapter aims to describe the assessment, treatment and modes of administration of nutrition and its impact on the outcome of head and neck cancer patients.

Chapter 3 – Nutritional counseling by RD has demonstrated that improves the quality of life through nutrient intake in hospitalized patients. In the last decades the role of registered dietitians (RD) has evolved including new responsibilities, activities and areas of work.

Between these, it is the integration of RD in nutrition support teams, with other professionals as physicians, pharmacists and nurses. One of the major roles of these teams is improving the safety and effectiveness of Parenteral Nutrition, therefore RD knowledge is of great interest in the management of critically ill patients. RD attends daily rounds, manage complex nutrition therapies and participate in policy and protocol development, perform research, feedback and education to other professionals. Other activities of RD is to document in the patient`s progress notes recommendations to the attending physician and bring information about: anthropometrics, fluid status, amount of nutrition received and estimated nutrition needs.

There are some settings, where RD has been granted privileges for order writing. Thus leading to greater assurance that an intervention will occur, improving nutritional status, better glycemic, caloric and electrolytic control as well as reduction in inappropriate parenteral nutritional use and cost savings.

Therefore, RD has to continue to integrate and expand their role in the management of parenteral nutrition, in Intensive Care Units (UCI) and in less critical patients who are taking artificial nutrition.

Chapter 4 – Parenteral nutrition associated liver disease (PNALD) is one of the most common complications of neonatal parenteral nutrition, yet much of its pathogenesis and treatment remains a mystery. In infants, this disease encompasses a spectrum of hepatobiliary changes including both cholestasis and fibrosis; but not generally steatosis. The earliest stage is often signaled by a serum direct bilirubin of >2mg/dL (>34μmol/L) while dependent on parenteral nutrition (PN). If the child remains reliant on PN, the cholestasis may progress to portal hypertension, cirrhosis, and eventually end-stage liver disease. Although a definitive treatment for PNALD does not exist, considerable research on the topic has been conducted, thus a review of the literature is the first step to better understand this illness.

In the following chapter the authors outline the history and incidence of this disease, beginning with the first reporting in the early 1970s to its current presence in modern neonatal intensive care units. They then explore the multiple factors believed to contribute to PNALD, including immature neonatal handling of bile (especially in those born premature) and a lack of enteral stimulation seen in those infants solely dependent on PN. Other factors such as sepsis and related inflammatory insults are examined. The authors explore recent studies implicating pro-inflammatory omega-6 fatty acids and the resulting encouraging trials with omega-3 fatty acids. Lastly, the authors discuss other damaging components of PN, including concerns about contaminants such as aluminum.

For each of the above mentioned theories of pathogenesis, multiple treatment methods have been proposed and attempted, but none alone has eliminated this disease. It is apparent that this multi-factorial issue will require a multi-faceted approach. The authors examine many of the attempted treatments and summarize their effectiveness, concluding with the most widely used and effective treatment regimes.

Chapter 5 – Parenteral nutrition-associated liver disease (PNALD) has been common in patients who require long-term parenteral nutrition (PN), it occurs in 15%-40% of adults receiving home PN and 40%-60% of infants receiving long-term PN for intestinal failure (IF). Clinical diagnosis of PNALD includes biochemical markers for liver disease, such as aspartate aminotransferase (AST), alanine aminotransferase (ALT), total bilirubin (TB), direct bilirubin (DB), and ruling out all other potential causes of liver disease. Meanwhile, liver biopsy is needed to definitively diagnose PNALD. The pathogenesis of PNALD is multifactorial and remains unclear. Risk factors include disruption of the enterohepatic circulation of bile acids, intestinal stasis with subsequent bacterial overgrowth, bile sludging with subsequent bile duct obstruction, early and/or recurrent central venous catheter-related sepsis, and nutrient deficiency or excess.

There is no specific treatment. Management strategies for its prevention and treatment depend on an understanding of many risk factors, and in general include consideration of early enteral feeding, the use of specialized lipid emulsions such as fish oil emulsions, and isolated small intestinal or combined liver-intestinal transplantation.

Chapter 6 – Refeeding syndrome is a well-described state of the series of metabolic and biochemical changes that occur during the supplemental feeding of malnourished patients. The shifts in fluids and electrolytes can lead to complications during artificial feeding and if not recognized and untreated can lead to death. Although the physiology and pathophysiology is well known, the circumstances under which the syndrome appears, clinical manifestations and management of these patients is less clear. To date, there are no published randomized controlled studies for refeeding syndrome in pediatric population. Published studies are generally lower level of evidence (level 3 and 4) that include cohort studies, case reports and expert opinions.

After the brief report of pathophysiology, the authors described refeeding syndrome cases from their clinical practice. Mainly, occurrence in pediatric patients has been reported in children with cancer. Then follow the patients with primary gastroenterological or neurological disease in the intensive care unit. In this chapter the authors describe risk assessment by defining the degree of malnutrition and planning of nutrition support. Baseline biochemical tests and laboratory monitoring, using reference change value of the most important analytes, can identify refeeding syndrome before symptoms appear. In this regard, the refeeding syndrome is laboratory diagnoses that provide a signal for treatment that is significantly simplified and includes termination of feeding, correction of electrolytes and continuation of feeding gradually and slowly.

In: Parenteral Nutrition
Editor: Shana Lelio

ISBN: 978-1-63321-112-4

Chapter 1

Parenteral Nutrition: Policies and Procedures, Safe Practices and Potential

Monica Habib, MS, RD, LD, CNSC, Leslie Shaw, RD, LD, CNSC, and Abdullah Shatnawei*[*]*, M.D., CNSC
Cleveland Clinic Foundation, Cleveland, Ohio, US

Abstract

Parenteral nutrition (PN) is the feeding modality of choice for patients with non-functional gastrointestinal (GI) tracts who are unable to maintain their nutrition and hydration enterally. Although it is a lifesaving therapy, it is associated with serious complications. A specialized nutrition support team can help select patients who are appropriate for parenteral nutrition. There are short term and long term indications for TPN. Short-term indications include ileus, tube feeding intolerance, small bowel obstruction, bowel rest and perioperative. Long-term indications include short bowel syndrome, recurrent small bowel obstructions, intestinal fistulae, gastrointestinal dysmotility, mesenteric ischemia, inflammatory bowel disease and radiation enteritis.

[*] Corresponding author email: shatnaa@ccf.org.

Once the patient is selected and a medical plan is made, appropriate intravenous access should be placed. For those requiring short-term parenteral nutrition, peripheral intravenous access is reasonable, however it is preferred to administer parenteral nutrition through a central vein. Central venous access can be gained via peripherally inserted central catheter, central venous catheter, tunneled catheter or med port. Short-term complications of parenteral nutrition include catheter related infections, catheter related thrombosis and deep vein thrombosis, abnormal blood sugars and electrolytes, fluid overload or dehydration. Long-term complications include parenteral nutrition induced liver disease, metabolic bone disease, catheter related infections and sepsis, mechanical complications of central catheters, and catheter thrombosis and blood clots. These complications can be minimized and sometimes prevented if managed by a specialized nutrition support team or a team with good knowledge about parenteral nutrition both in the inpatient and outpatient settings.

Parenteral nutrition (PN) is the feeding modality of choice for patients with non-functional gastrointestinal (GI) tracts who are unable to maintain their nutrition and hydration enterally. Parenteral nutrition is a complex therapy involving the intravenous infusion of macro and micronutrients directly into the bloodstream for optimal absorption. The main components of parenteral formulas include dextrose, amino acids and lipids. Although PN is a lifesaving therapy for many patients, it is associated with serious short and long-term complications that can be life-threatening. Therefore, selection of the appropriate patient for parenteral therapy is crucial.

Indications for PN include:

- Paralytic ileus
- Small bowel obstruction
- Intestinal ischemia
- High output GI fistula
- Short bowel syndrome or severe malabsorption
- Radiation enteritis
- Intestinal dysmotility or chronic pseudo-obstruction
- Severe acute necrotizing pancreatitis
- Severe GI bleed
- Graft-versus-host disease requiring bowel rest
- Tube feeding failure or lack of enteral access

- Pre-operative nutrition support (in severely malnourished patients, for a minimum of 7-10 days)

Selection and management of PN patients should be the responsibility of a multidisciplinary Nutrition Support Team (NST), consisting of registered dietitians, nurses, pharmacists and physicians. Consults received by the NST should be evaluated for PN appropriateness, using nutritional status information, pertinent diagnoses and rationale and/or indication for intravenous feeding. After evaluation by the NST, the ideal nutrition support therapy can be recommended. Implementation of a formal PN approval process has been shown to decrease total and inappropriate use of PN in the hospital setting, as well as PN related complications, such as catheter sepsis and mechanical problems [1,2]. In addition to providing patients with the most beneficial nutrition support therapy, use of NST will help with cost containment, as PN is a more expensive therapy compared to enteral nutrition [3]. Members of a Nutrition Support Team can also provide continuing education to medical staff regarding nutrition support [3].

Once a patient is approved for PN, existing IV access should be evaluated. If IV access has not been established, selection of the appropriate catheter is key. For patients requiring a short course of PN (less than 2 weeks), a peripheral IV is acceptable for use, though only peripheral PN (PPN) can be infused. Peripheral IVs require frequent IV site rotations (at least every 48 to 72 hours), as PN is a hyperosmolar infusate and increases the risk of phlebitis [4]. It is recommended to keep the osmolarity of PPN at or below 900 mOsm/L. As dextrose and amino acids are the major contributors to PN osmolarity, total calories may be limited. A typical PPN solution contains 150-300 grams of dextrose and 50-100 grams of protein [4]. Lipids are normally used to provide additional calories. However, greater PPN volume allows for greater concentrations of greater dextrose and amino acids. The ideal patient for PPN is one that has good peripheral venous access, can tolerate large volumes of fluid and is not severely malnourished [4]. Patients that are severely malnourished, have poor venous access or are on a fluid restriction are better served with a central solution [4].

Midline catheters should be considered when PPN therapy is expected to continue for more than 6 days [5]. Midline catheters are peripheral catheters, between 20 and 25 cm in length, that are inserted in the superficial veins of the antecubital area and do not extend past the axillary vein [5]. Placement can be done at the bedside, using ultrasound guidance. Midline catheters can stay in place for approximately 2 to 6 weeks, though still carry a risk for thrombophlebitis [5,6]. Prevention of peripheral vein thrombophlebitis can be accomplished by practicing aseptic technique during catheter placement and care, choosing a smaller gauge catheter made of polyurethane or silicone, ensuring appropriate solution osmolarity, using lipid based solutions, keeping the pH between 5 and 9 and adequately fixing the catheter in place to prevent movement or dislodgement [5]. Midlines are not the first choice catheters for PN infusion.

For patients whose needs cannot be met using PPN, central parenteral nutrition (CPN) should be initiated. CPN is infused via a central vein, allowing for larger concentrations of nutrient components and essentially unlimited osmolarity. CPN requires a venous access device (VAD) with tip placement in a large diameter central vein. This enables the hypertonic PN solution to be rapidly diluted in order to avoid irritating the vein wall [7]. Optimal tip position for a VAD is near the junction of the superior vena cava (SVC) and the right atrium [8]. Any tip located in the upper third of the SVC or abutting the vein wall is not ideal for CPN infusion [8]. VADs with tips located in the proximal third of the SVC and above are significantly more likely to develop a venous thrombosis versus those with tips in the distal third of the SVC or below [9]. Catheters near the SVC/right atrial junction are also less likely to experience malfunctions, such as infusion difficulties or withdrawal occlusions [10].

The Nutrition Support Team clinician should work closely with patients and their primary services in order to select the appropriate VAD, with close consideration of the advantages and disadvantages for each device, as well as, the estimated length of time PN therapy will be required [11]. Tunneled catheter are more appropriate for long-term use, whereas non-tunneled catheters are more suitable for short-term use, such as in an acute care setting [6]. The necessary number of catheter lumens should also be assessed, as patients are often receiving supplemental IV fluids and medications, such as antibiotics, in addition to CPN. Single lumen catheters are preferred, as infection risk increases with greater number of lumens [12]. If possible, CPN should be cycled (or infused over a period of less than 24 hours) to allow for other infusions and ease of blood draws. In addition, attention should be paid to the material from which the catheter is made, in order to ensure the safety of ethanol lock therapy, if available to the patient. Ethanol locks cannot be used in catheters made from polyurethane due to the risk of catheter degradation. Finally, the clinician must consider the patient or caregiver's physical ability to care for the VAD, cognitive function, body image concerns and most favorable exit site location prior to placement. The NST clinician can mark the preferred exit site location, making sure to avoid wounds, skin folds, previous catheter sites, and clothing pieces that may irritate or contaminate the catheter [11].

Short-term Central Catheters

Non-tunneled catheters are frequently used in the acute care setting for short-term PN therapy (days to weeks). Access is typically obtained percutaneously via the subclavian, jugular, femoral or antecubital route. Sutures are placed at the exit site, as well as a sterile dressing, to prevent dislodgement [6]. Short-term non-tunneled catheters can have multiple lumens and are designed for continuous use. It is not appropriate to send a patient home with a short-term catheter.

Medium-term Central Catheters

Peripherally inserted central catheters (PICCs) are non-tunneled and are inserted into the antecubital vessels (basilic, brachial and cephalic) [6]. PICC lines are used in the acute and home setting. Placement can be done at the bedside by specially trained medical staff or in the Interventional Radiology suite. In terms of home parenteral nutrition (HPN), PICC lines are recommended for patients that are anticipated to require less than 60 days of therapy [8]. Advantages of PICCs include decreased risk of thoracic complications (due to the antecubital placement approach), low placement costs and ease of removal [5, 6]. Disadvantages include ease of dislodgement or obstruction and limits to self-care due to one arm being disabled [5]. Hohn catheters are similar to PICCs in that they are non-tunneled and for medium-term use, however, Hohn catheters are inserted into a central vein.

Long-term Central Catheters

Tunneled cuffed catheters or implanted ports are recommended for patients who require long-term PN (greater than 3 months). Popular brands of tunneled cuffed catheters include Hickman, Groshong and Broviac. Tunneled cuffed catheters are typically placed in an Interventional Radiology suite via the subclavian or jugular vessels [6]. Catheter tunneling is thought to decrease infection risk by separating the exit and venipuncture sites of the catheter, however, rigorous aseptic nursing care has been deemed the most significant factor in reducing catheter infections [13]. Advantages of these catheters include decreased risk of dislodgement and ease of self-care [6]. Implanted ports are placed subcutaneously, therefore require the patient to access the port daily using a Huber needle. While this may make the implanted port less attractive to patients requiring daily PN therapy, some patients prefer a port due to the minimal alteration in their body image [11].

There are several additional factors that should be considered when choosing or evaluating a patient's VAD. The tip of the VAD should terminate in the superior vena cava (SVC)/right atrium (RA) junction or slightly inside the right atrium in order to avoid catheter malfunctions, including withdrawal occlusions or difficulty infusing [10]. Most significantly, tip position can affect the risk of catheter thrombosis in patients receiving high osmolarity PN. VADs with tips terminating in the proximal SVC are more likely to develop venous thrombosis when compared to VADs with tips terminating in the distal third of the SVC or lower [9]. Tip position can be confirmed during placement or post-placement by obtaining a chest X-ray [5]. As catheters can have multiple lumens, it is also important for patients to receive only the number of lumens necessary for their IV therapy. Managing more than one lumen long-term increases infection risk [12]. PN should be cycled to allow for other medications, such as IV antibiotics, to be given when the PN is off. If multiple catheter lumens are needed, patients should be trained to dedicate one specific lumen to PN therapy [11]. Lastly, ethanol lock therapy (ELT) should be provided to patients with silicone catheters. ELT is bactericidal and fungicidal and has been shown to decrease infection rates in HPN patients [14]. Ethanol is instilled into the catheter lumen using a pre-filled syringe while PN is not infusing. The ethanol then dwells in the lumen until PN is ready to be infused, where it is then flushed through the catheter. It is not recommended to use ETL with polyurethane catheters, as there is a known chemical reaction between ethanol and polyurethane and the physical properties of the catheter may be impacted posing a concern for catheter degradation.

Initiating Parenteral Nutrition

Once a patient is determined to have an appropriate indication for PN, electrolytes, fluid balance and nutrition status should be evaluated. Patients that are malnourished are at risk for refeeding syndrome, which refers to metabolic and physiologic shifts of fluid, electrolytes and minerals that occur as a result of aggressive nutrition support [15]. Dextrose delivery stimulates insulin secretion, which causes an intracellular shift of electrolytes resulting in hypophosphatemia, hypomagnesemia and hypokalemia. Edema, cardiac arrhythmia and hemolysis are severe complications of refeeding syndrome [15]. Patients who are deemed at risk for refeeding syndrome should have their electrolytes repleted prior to initiation of PN therapy. Low calories should be provided initially, with slow advancement to goal.

The first bag of PN should contain the patient's goal protein and half of their estimated energy needs or 150 to 200 grams of dextrose. Blood glucose should be monitored every 6 hours [16]. Electrolytes should be monitored daily and repleted as needed prior to increasing dextrose calories to goal. Protein restriction is rarely required. Lipids should be provided in order to prevent essential fatty acid deficiency (EFAD). In order to avoid EFAD, 2 to 4% of total calories should be provided as linoleic acid and 0.25 to 0.5% of total calories as alpha-linolenic acid [17]. This can be accomplished by providing 1000 calories of soy-based lipids weekly [18]. When determining the appropriate starting volume for PN, the patient's current fluid balance, intakes and outputs and co-morbidities/disease state should be considered. There are multiple existing equations to estimate fluid requirements. Overall, the goal should be to maintain adequate urine output and electrolytes and replace insensible and measured losses. Fluid may need to be restricted in patients with heart failure or renal failure requiring dialysis.

Safe Practices

PN is a complex admixture containing multiple components that can cause serious harm or death if improperly prepared or administered [17]. The PN order form should be well organized and easy to understand. Mandatory components of the PN order form include: type of venous access (central or peripheral), height, weight, diagnosis, indication for PN, contact number for reference person and prescriber, hang time guidelines, information regarding potential incompatibilities and warning mechanism for excessive rate of nutrient administration [17,19]. It is not mandatory, but strongly recommended to include the following items on the PN order form: nutrient dosing guidelines based on weight and age, recommended nutrient ranges, guidelines to assist in nutrient and volume calculations, monitoring guidelines, guidelines for stopping or interrupting the PN infusion, specific content of multivitamin and trace element preparations, specific amino acid and IVFE brands available and insulin guidelines [19]. When considering the actual PN label, base components, electrolytes, micronutrients and medications are required to be written as amount per day. The dosing weight of the patient is also required [17].

Electronic medical charting and order writing is considered optimal for PN patients. An electronic PN order form can be designed to alert the prescriber to incompatibilities or errors in the PN formulation prior to signing. The order form should also be able to be edited daily based on the patient's clinical status. An electronic PN ordering system can also be used to keep prescribers informed of drug shortages and acceptable substitutions available at their institution. Ideally, the orders should be reviewed by a well-trained, PN therapy designated pharmacist. The pharmacist and the prescribers should have an open line of communication to discuss errors or miscalculations in the PN order if identified. In addition, the pharmacist can notify the prescriber of any PN orders that are not received, in order to assure that patients do not miss their daily PN therapy due to an oversight.

Electrolyte Abnormalities

Electrolyte requirements vary depending on the patient's current underlying disease, electrolyte, renal, and fluid status. Electrolyte abnormalities can result from excess intake or losses, intracellular shifts, and/or fluid imbalances. Electrolytes are added to the PN solutions in amounts sufficient to provide for daily needs. The most common electrolyte abnormalities include sodium, potassium, calcium, magnesium phosphorus and acid-base balance.

Sodium is a major extracellular cation and functions in the maintenance of osmotic pressure and in acid–base balance. The usual dose is 1 to 2 mEq/kg per day [20]. Requirements may be increased when there are excess losses from urine, stoma, or fistulae or decreased in renal, cardiac, or hepatic failure. Hyponatremia is the most common electrolyte abnormality which results from impaired renal excretion of water in the setting of continuous water intake. The symptoms of mild hyponatremia (serum sodium <125mEq/L) include nausea, weakness, lethargy and muscle cramps [21]. If hyponatremia develops quickly more serious symptoms such as seizures, permanent brain damage, respiratory arrest and death, may occur. To help treat hyponatremia with the use of PN, the clinician should either concentrate the formula or increase the sodium content, not exceeding 154mEq/L. The following equation is commonly used to calculate sodium deficit. The rate of correction should not exceed 8 to 12 mMol/L/d. [22]

Sodium Deficit (mEq) = 0.6 x Weight in kg x [140-Plasma Sodium] [22]

Hypernatremia is usually caused by excess water loss, such as diarrhea, fever, osmotic diuresis diabetes insipidous or simply a hypertonic solution. Symptoms are similar to those of hyponatremia. Hypernatremia is treated by replacing water. The following equation is calculated to safely correct hypernatremia.

Water Deficit (L) = 0.6 X Weight in kg x [(Serum Sodium/140)-1][22]

Potassium is the major cation of intracellular fluid. The normal dose is 1 to 2 mEq per kg or approximately 60-120mEq/d [20]. Where the PN solution should provide maintenance potassium requirements, acute deficits should be corrected with an IV replacement dose. Generally mild hypokalemia can be treated in the next bag of PN. If there is severe hypokalemia, it should be treated with either oral replacements, which is preferred, or IV replacements. Intravenous replacements should be given in increments of 20mEq over a one hour infusion. Please see Table 1 for treatment of hypokalemia. Hypokalemia may result from losses in urine or the GI tract such as diuretic therapy, nasogastric suction, vomiting or diarrhea. Symptoms include weakness, malaise, fatigue, paralysis, constipation, ileus and heart arrhythmias. [21]

Hyperkalemia can be caused by medications such as cyclosporine and tacrolimus [21]. Symptoms include twitching, cramping, weakness, and heart arrhythmias. In mild cases of hyperkalemia, simply decrease or omit potassium in the next bag. In case of severe hyperkalemia (>6.5mEq/L), discontinue the PN bag and treat by IV calcium, sodium bicarbonate, insulin, dextrose or beta-agonist [21]. The combination of the above therapy helps to move potassium intracellularly and restore normal membrane excitability.

Table 1. Treating hypokalemia

Serum Potassium	Calculation of Deficit	Replacement Dose
3-3.5 mMol/L	100-200mEq	½ K deficit. Prefer to replace orally if possible.
2.5-3 mMol/L	150-250mEq	20mEq in 100mL NS over 1hr if <3.5. Re-check 2 hrs after replacement and repeat as needed.
2-2.5mMol/L	200-300mEq	20mEq in 100mL NS over 1hr if <3.5. Re-check 2 hrs after replacement and repeat as needed.

Sodium and potassium are added in the form of chloride or acetate salts. Chloride is a major extracellular anion and functions in the maintenance of osmotic pressure and acid–base balance. Acetate maybe added to PN solutions when clinically appropriate since it is converted to bicarbonate in the liver and functions as a systemic base. Bicarbonate should not be added to PN solutions as it is not compatible with other additives and may form a precipitate.

Calcium is an extracellular cation that is essential for normal muscle contraction, nerve function, blood coagulation, and bone mineralization. Calcium levels are maintained via parathyroid hormone (PTH), vitamin D and calcitonin. The usual dose is 10 to 15 mEq per day [20]. Sixty percent of serum calcium is bound to protein, primarily albumin. Therefore in the presence of a low serum albumin level, a low serum calcium level needs to be adjusted for hypoalbuminemia. This equation provides an estimate of the adjusted calcium level in the presence of hypoalbuminemia. When in doubt and when the serum albumin is less than 2.8 grams per dL, an ionized calcium level should be obtained.

Corrected Total Calcium (mg/dL) = Measured Total Ca (mg/dL) + 0.8 x [4.0 - Serum Albumin(g/dL)][23]

Hypocalcemia can result from hypoparathyroidism, acute pancreatitis, vitamin D deficiency hyperphosphatemia and/or respiratory alkalosis [23]. Medications such as calcitonin, bisphosphates and furosemide can also cause hypocalcemia. Symptoms of hypocalcemia include hypotension, muscle cramps, tetany and seizures [21]. If repletion dose is needed after adjusting for albumin, 7 to 14mEq of IV Calcium gluconate should be given over 2 to 4 hours, where 1 gm provides 4.65 mEq of calcium. Hypercalcemia often occurs with bone metastases and hyperparathyroidism which causes bone resorbtion [23]. The symptoms of hypercalcemia include nausea, vomiting, anorexia, muscle weakness, confusion and heart arrhythmias [21]. The underlying cause of hypercalcemia should be identified and treated. Mild hypercalcemia can be treated by removing or decreasing calcium and ensuring adequate hydration is being given. In the case of severe hypercalcemia, IV hydration, furosemide and/or bisphosphonates may be given [21].

Along with calcium, phosphorus is the major component of bone hydroxyapatite and teeth. Phosphorus is the primary intracellular anion and functions in the metabolism of carbohydrate, fat, and protein. The usual dose is 20 to 40 mMol per day [20]. Hypophosphatemia can be the result of increased excretion, or aluminum containing antacids. Mild hypophosphatemia can be treated with increased phosphorus in the next bag, where as severe hypophosphatemia should be repleted with administration of IV sodium phosphorus (NaPO4) or potassium phosphorus (KPO4) [21].

Table 2. Treatment of Hypophosphatemia

Serum Phosphorus (mg/dL)	Repletion Dose
2.3-3 mg/dL	0.32 mMol/kg NaPO4 or KPO4 over 4-6 hrs
1.6-2.2 mg/dL	0.64 mMol/kg NaPO4 or KPO4 over 4-6 hrs
≤1.5 mg/dL	1mMol/kg over 8-12 hrs of NaPO4 if ≥K 4 mEq/L

Hyperphosphatemia can occur when there is cellular destruction from hypercatabolism, hemolysis, or trauma. The symptoms seen with hyperphosphatemia are due to resulting hypocalcemia [21]

The combination of calcium and phosphorus in PN formulas has the potential of forming a precipitate. Thus, the maximum calcium and phosphorus product should be < 200 in a PN formula as per the formula below.

Calcium-Phosphorus Product= mEq Ca/L x mEq PO4/L [24]

Magnesium functions in enzyme reactions such as glycolysis and in all reactions involving adenosine triphosphate (ATP). Magnesium is often depleted in patients with protein calorie malnutrition and prolonged IV fluid therapy. The usual dose of magnesium sulfate is 8 to 20 mEq per day [20]. Hypomagnesemia is a result of excessive GI or renal losses, or redistribution of the intracellular fluid compartment. Many medications can cause hypomagnesemia as well, which is a very common occurrence in hospitalized patient. Symptoms of hypomagnesemia include muscle weakness, tetany, convulsions, nausea, vomiting and apathy [21]. Treatment of hypomagnesemia can be done by either increasing magnesium in the next bag or giving IV repletion. Magnesium sulfate provides 8.12 mEq per gram of magnesium. Hypermagnesemia can be caused by renal failure, hypothyroidism, trauma, rhabdomyolysis or dehydration. Symptoms include neurological, neuromuscular or cardiac abnormalities. Treatment of mild hypermagnesemia is to decrease magnesium in the next bag while treatment of severe hypermagnesemia includes IV calcium and hemodialysis [21]. Vitamins, minerals, and trace elements are added daily to the PN solution in order to prevent deficiencies. Parenteral vitamins and trace elements are given as standard multiple-vitamin and trace element preparations. In the event that vitamin, mineral, or trace element deficiencies or unusual losses occur, they can sometimes be supplemented above the amount normally added to the PN solution. Recently, in the United States there have been national shortages of these trace elements, namely zinc. Table 3 illustrates symptoms of trace element deficiencies.

Table 3. Symptoms of Trace Element Deficiencies [25, 26]

Trace Element	Normal Serum Value	Symptoms of deficiency
Zinc	50-150mcg/L	Dermatitis, impaired wound healing, diarrhea, hyogeusia
Copper	70-150mcg/L	Hypochromic microcytic anemia, neutropenia
Chromium	1-3mg/mL	Glucose intolerance, peripheral neuropathy, insulin resistance
Manganese	2-3mcg/dL	Dermatitis, nausea, vomiting
Selenium	0.01-0.34mcg/dL	Cardiomyopathy

Metabolic Complications

Hyperglycemia is the most common adverse effect of PN and is associated with increased morbidity and mortality in hospitalized patients. Close monitoring of blood sugars along with aggressive treatment reduces hyperglycemia and improves outcomes. Blood sugars in hospitalized patients receiving PN should be maintained between 140- 180 mg/dL [27]. Capillary blood glucose levels should be monitored every 6 hours until adequately controlled. PN-associated hyperglycemia may be treated by insulin drip, short- or long acting insulin administered subcutaneously, insulin added to the PN or a combination of these methods. For known diabetic patients, 0.1 units of regular human insulin per 1 gram of dextrose can be used as a starting dose [28]. If hyperglycemia persists beyond 0.3 units of insulin per 1 gram of dextrose, an insulin drip should be considered [28]. In some instances it may be necessary to reduce dextrose calories and replace with lipid calories to aid in blood glucose control.

Hypoglycemia, defined as a blood glucose concentration of <70mg/dL, may occur if an excessive amount of insulin is added to the PN solution or within 15 to 30 minutes after abrupt discontinuation of PN infusion [29]. To avoid these problems, insulin should be added in increments to the PN solution and blood sugars monitored frequently until the appropriate dose is determined. To prevent rebound hypoglycemia, PN infusions should be tapered down over a period of 1-to-2 hours prior to discontinuation to allow for serum insulin adaptation [30].

Non-infectious Catheter Complications

In patients with central access, heparin-induced thrombocytopenia (HIT), a severe immune-mediated adverse reaction that occurs by intravascular platelet aggregation, can develop into arterial and venous thrombus [31]. Catheter occlusions, which cause the inability to infuse or aspirate blood, can also occur. When a complete occlusion occurs, fluid cannot be instilled and blood cannot be aspirated out. Whereas in an incomplete occlusion, fluid can be infused however, blood cannot be aspirated. A venous thrombus can occur if the catheter tip is malpostitioned. It is recommended that the tip of the catheter be placed in the superior vena cava adjacent to the right atrium. In the case of a tunneled catheter such a Hickman, a tunneled catheter breakage is a risk. This must be repaired as soon as possible to prevent air embolism and leakage of blood. An air embolism, although rare, is a potentially fatal complication where either during or after insertion, there is catheter breakage or a disconnection of caps. Catheter dislodgement can occur with any CVC and move out of central circulation in which case the catheter should be replaced. Pinch-off syndrome refers to the compression of the subclavian vein catheter between the clavicle and first rib resulting in a catheter obstruction [32]. An indication of pinch off syndrome is if there is a relief of the compression when the arm is elevated.

Septic (Infectious) Complications

Sepsis can occur during CPN infusion therefore, if there is a sudden change in the patient's usual temperature, new onset shaking chills, leukocytosis, or unexplained hyperglycemia, the CVC should be viewed as the possible source of infection. This is known as a catheter-related blood stream infection (CRBSI). In a temporary CVC, if there is no other obvious source of infection the line should be removed and re-sited [33]. A long-term CVC may be treated in situ providing the patient's symptoms improve after antibiotic treatment is started. The catheter must be removed if yeast or Staphylococcus coli are cultured [33].

Discharging with PN

Home parenteral nutrition (HPN), is the provision of intravenous dextrose, amino acids, lipids, electrolytes, vitamins, minerals, trace elements and fluids to maintain nutritional status in the home setting. In order to safely discharge a patient on HPN, a thorough evaluation and appropriate preparation must be completed. One must initially determine the indication for HPN is appropriate. The patients indicated for HPN are those who are unable to maintain nutrition status orally due to short bowel syndrome, radiation enteritis, high output fistula or stoma, bowel obstruction or motility disorders. Next is to determine the length of therapy and the end point of care, as this will aide in determining the appropriate type of central venous access.

It is essential that a multidisciplinary team be involved with the decision making process. Case management, social work, nurses and dietitians should be notified of plans for discharging. The case managers verify insurance benefits for HPN coverage which may include home nursing visits, HPN training or sub-acute, rehabilitation or long term facility placements. Social workers will assess the level of function of the patient, ability to cope, family support and safety in the home. Nurses will educate the patient and family member's catheter care and HPN procedures such as operation of the infusion pump, PN set up and disconnect and maintenance of input and output. The dietitian will perform the nutritional assessment, establish calorie and protein needs and determine goal weight.

Once this is completed and the patients' formula is stable with fluids, electrolytes and goal calories, the PN will be cycled by decreasing infusion time by 4 to 6 hours per day for 2 to 3 days. Decreasing infusion time allows the liver to mobilize stored glycogen, promotes nitrogen retention and may decrease the incidence of fatty liver [34]. Cycling also allows for administration of other IV medications and allowing the patient time unencumbered by PN. However, cycling put the patient at increased risk of hyperglycemia and volume overload since the same nutrients are infused over a shorter time period, hence why clinicians should gradually decrease in the infusion time over a period of 2 to 3 days. The rate of infusion at the beginning and end should be tapered or ramped up and down respectively as to avoid hyper- or hypoglycemia.

Once discharged, the patient should follow up as an outpatient in order to manage possible complications. Routine lab work should be obtained weekly then decreased once the formula is stabilized. Trace elements should be taken every 3-6 months and phospholipid fatty acid annually to avoid deficiencies.

Long Term Complications of HPN

Metabolic Bone Disease (MBD)

MBD is seen in long term PN patients yet the etiology is unknown. Possible causes include inadequate calcium due to calcium and phosphorus losses from acidosis or urinary losses, as well as excess amino acids, cyclic infusions, metabolic acidosis, vitamin D deficiency, copper deficiency and aluminum contamination [35]. Aluminum exceeding 5 mcg/kg/day may be associated with bone toxicity. Providing 10 to 15 mEq of calcium, 20 to 40 mMol of phosphorus and 15mEq of magnesium can help minimize these effects [35]. Monitor signs of MDB such as loss of height, bone or back pain.

Obtain 24 hour urine collection for calcium and magnesium ever y 6 to 12 months and adjust in PN to maintain positive balance. Those patients who are at risk should undergo a dual x-ray absorptiometry (DXA) scan every 1 to 2 years.

Liver Disease

Liver dysfunction is common in patients receiving long term PN which can progress to PN-associated liver disease (PNALD). Complicated PNALD includes extensive portal fibrosis or cirrhosis, bilirubin ≥3.5mg/Dl for ≥1 month, ascites, portal hypertension, hepatic encephalopathy, or factor V concentration <50% [36]. Although it is of unclear etiology, there are ways to decrease risk of liver function abnormalities in long term PN patients including avoiding overfeeding, preventing EFAD, and cycling PN.

Transition from PN to EN

Enteral nutrition remains the preferred route of nutrition therefore as gastrointestinal function returns, the patient should be transitioned to enteral nutrition by tube or oral nutrition. When oral intake approximates 50% of a patient's needs PN can be discontinued.

References

[1] Maurer J, Weinbaum F, Turner J, et al. Reducing the Inappropriate Use of Parenteral Nutrition in an Acute Care Teaching Hospital. *JPEN-Parenter Enter.* 1996; 20:272-274.

[2] Nehme, AE. Nutritional Support of the Hospitalized Patient. *JAMA-J Am Med Assoc.* 1980; 243:1906-1908.

[3] O'Brien DD, Hodges RE, Day AT, Waxman KS, Rebello T. Recommendations of Nutrition Support Team Promote Cost Containment. *JPEN-Parenter Enter.* 1986; 10:300-302.

[4] Mirtallo JM, Patel M. Overview of Parenteral Nutrition. In: Mueller CM, ed. *The A.S.P.E.N. Adult Nutrition Support Core Curriculum.* 2nd

ed. Silver Spring, MD: American Society for Parenteral and Enteral Nutrition; 2012:234-244.

[5] Pittiruti M, Hamilton H, Biffi R, MacFie J, Pertkiewicz M. ESPEN Guidelines on Parenteral Nutrition: Central Venous Catheters (access, care, diagnosis and therapy of complications). *Clin Nutr.* 2009; 28:365-377.

[6] Krzywda EA, Andris DA, Edmiston CE. Parenteral Access Devices. In: Mueller CM, ed. *The A.S.P.E.N. Adult Nutrition Support Core Curriculum.* 2nd ed. Silver Spring, MD: American Society for Parenteral and Enteral Nutrition; 2012:265-283.

[7] Steiger E. Vascular Access for Parenteral Nutrition. In: DeLegge MH, ed. Nutrition and Gastrointestinal Disease. Totowa NJ: Humana Press; 2008:290.

[8] Steiger E, HPEN Working Group. Consensus Statements Regarding Optimal Management of Home Parenteral Nutrition (HPN) Access. *JPEN-Parenter Enter.* 2006; 30:S94-S95.

[9] Cadman A, Lawrance JAL, Fitzsimmons L, Spencer-Shaw A, Swindell R. To clot or not to clot? That is the question in central venous catheters. *Clin Radiol.* 2004; 56:349-355.

[10] Petersen J, Delaney JH, Brakstad MT, Rowbotham RK, Bagley Jr CM. Silicone venous access devices positioned with their tips high in the superior vena cava are more likely to malfunction. *Am J Surg.* 1999; 178:38-41.

[11] Stafford JR, Emery DM. Getting the Patient Out of the Hospital on Parenteral Nutrition: Catheter Selection, Assessment, and Education. *Support Line.* 2007; 29(3):3-7.

[12] Henriques HF 3rd, Karmy-Jones R, Knoll SM, Copes WS, Giordano JM. Avoiding complications of long-term venous access. *Am Surg.* 1993; 59(9):555-558.

[13] Keohane PP, Attrill H, Northover J, et al. Effect of Catheter Tunneling and a Nutrition Nurse on Catheter Sepsis During Parenteral Nutrition: A Controlled Trial. *Lancet.* 1983; 322:1388-1390.

[14] John BK, Khan MA, Speerhas R, et al. Ethanol Lock Therapy in Reducing Catheter-Related Bloodstream Infections in Adult Home Parenteral Nutrition Patients: Results of a Retrospective Study. *JPEN-Parenter Enter.* 2012; 36:603-610.

[15] Solomon SM, Kirby DK. The Refeeding Syndrome: A Review. *JPEN-Parenter Enter.* 1990; 14(1):90-97.

[16] Kumpf VJ, Gervasio J. Complications of Parenteral Nutrition. In: Mueller CM, ed. *The A.S.P.E.N. Adult Nutrition Support Core Curriculum.* 2nd ed. Silver Spring, MD: American Society for Parenteral and Enteral Nutrition; 2012:285-297.

[17] Mirtallo J, Canada T, Johnson D, et al. Safe Practices for Parenteral Nutrition. *JPEN-Parenter Enter.* 2004; 28:S39-S70.

[18] Jeppesen PB, Hoy CE, Mortensen PB. Essential fatty acid deficiency in patients receiving home parenteral nutrition. *Am J Clin Nutr.* 1998; 68:126-133.

[19] Kumpf VJ, Mirtallo JM, Petersen C. Parenteral Nutrition Formulations: Preparation and Ordering. In: Merritt R, ed. *The A.S.P.E.N. Nutrition Support Practice Manual.* 2nd ed. Silver Spring, MD. American Society for Parenteral and Enteral Nutrition; 2005:97-107.

[20] Baumgartner TG. Clinical Guide to Parenteral Micronutrition. 3rd ed. Fujisawa USA; Deerfield, IL 1997.

[21] Brown RO, Dickerson RN. Drug-nutrient reactions. Am J Managed Care. 1999; 5:345-352.

[22] Whitmire SJ. Fluid,electrolytes, and acid-base balance. In: Matarese, LE, Gottschlich NM, ed. *Contemporary Nutrition Support Practice. A Clinical Guide.* 2nd ed. St. Louis, MO: WB Saunders; 2003; 122-144.

[23] Singer FR, Bethune JE, Massry SG. Hyercalcemia and hypokalemia. *Clin Nephro.* 1997; 7:154-162.

[24] Task force for the revision of safe practices for parenteral nutrition. Safe practices for parenteral nutrition. *JPEN J Parenter Enteral Nutr.* 2004; 28:S39-S70.

[25] Strausburg KT. Nutrition/metabolic assessment. In: Teasley-Strausburg K,ed. *Nutrition Support Handbook.* Cincinnati, OH:Harvey Whitney; 1992

[26] Jensen GL, Biakley J. Clinical manifestation of nutrient deficiency. *JPEN J Parenter Enteral Nutr.*2002; 26S:S29-233.

[27] McMahon MM et al. A.S.P.E.N. clinical guidelines: nutrition support of adult patients with hyperglycemia. *JPEN J Parenter Enteral Nutr.* 2013; 37(1):23-36.

[28] McCowen CK. Malhotra A Bistrian BR. Stress-induced hyperglycemia. *Crit Care Clin.*2001; 17:107-124.

[29] Wagman LP Miller KB Thomas RB Newsome HH, Weir GC. The effect of acute discontinuation of total parenteral nutrition. *Ann Surg.* 1986; 204:524-529.

[30] ASPEN Board of Directors and the Clinical Guidelines Task Force. Guidelines for the use of parenteral and enteral nutrition in adult and pediatric patients. *JPEN J Parenter Enteral Nutr.* 2002; 26(1 Suppl):1SA-138SA.

[31] Richardson DK. Practice, standard of care, and strategies to prevent infection: A review of flushing solutions and injection caps. *JAVA J Asso Vascular-Access.* 2007; 12(2):74-84.

[32] Andris DA, Krzywda EA. Catheter pinch-off syndrome: recognition and management. *J Intravenous Nurs.* 1997; 20:233-237.

[33] Maki DG. Line sepsis in the ICU:Prevention, diagnosis and management. *Semin Respir Crit Care Med.* 2003; 24:23-26.

[34] Maini B, Blackburn G, Bistrian BR et al. Cyclic hyperalimentation: An optimal technique for preservation of visceral protein. *J Surg Res.* 1976:20; 515-525.

[35] Hamilton C , Seidner DL. Metabolic bone disease and parenteral nutrition. *Curr Gastroentrol Rep.* 2004; 6(4):335-341.

[36] Cavicchi M Beau P Crenn P Degott C Messing B. Prevalence of liver disease and contributing factors in patients receiving home parenteral nutrition for permanent intestinal failure. *Ann Intern Med.* 2000; 132(7):525-532.

In: Parenteral Nutrition
Editor: Shana Lelio

ISBN: 978-1-63321-112-4

Chapter 2

Nutritional Considerations for Head and Neck Cancer Patients

***Ahmad Alshadwi*[*1], *BDS*,**
and Mohammed M. Nadershah*[†2], *BDS, MSc
[1]Resident, department of oral and maxillofacial surgery, Boston University, Boston Medical Center, Boston, MA, US
[2]Academic Faculty, King Abdulaziz University, Dental School, Jeddah, Saudi Arabia

Abstract

Approximately 35-60% of all head and neck cancer patients are malnourished at the time of their diagnosis, either due to tumor burden and obstruction of intake and/or the anorexia/cachexia associated with their cancer. Most of those patients will require parentral nutrition before and after surgical treatment, adjuvant chemotherapy, and/ or radiotherapy. Moreover, head and neck cancer generally affect older population with multiple medical comorbidities that may complicate managing their nutritional needs. Nutritional interventions should be initiated before the cancer treatment begins and these interventions need to be ongoing following completion of treatment to ensure optimal outcomes for patients. A nutritional assessment must be part of all

[*] Corresponding author: alshadwi@bu.edu; Tel. 617-414-4838, Fax. 617-414-4126.
[†] mnadershah@gmail.com.

comprehensive treatment plans for patients with head and neck cancer. Alternative nutritional interventions such as immune-enhancing nutrients or anti-cytokine pharmaceutical agents may also be effective as adjuvant therapies, but more research is needed to quantify their clinical effect. This chapter aims to describe the assessment, treatment and modes of administration of nutrition and its impact on the outcome of head and neck cancer patients.

Introduction

Localized and/or systemic head and neck cancer and its treatment modalities can seriously undermine a patient's nutritional status. Malnutrition and nutritional deficits have a significant negative impact on mortality, morbidity and quality of life [1]. Up to 57% of patients with head and neck cancer present with malnutrition with a greater than 10% weight loss from baseline body mass [2]. Moreover, head and neck cancers may cause significant trismus, odynophagia, dysphagia and aspiration. Large tumors can obstruct the aerodigestive system thereby exacerbating malnutrition. Moreover, treatment options for head and neck cancer include surgery, chemotherapy and radiation therapy. Each of these interventions has side effects that may further contribute to malnutrition [3].

Alcohol and tobacco use frequently exacerbates this problem [4, 5]. Alcohol is devoid of essential vitamins, proteins and fats but requires certain micronutrients to be metabolized, thus further depleting nutrient stores. Alcohol metabolites may actually contribute to cancer growth and further nutritional decay. The combination of alcohol and tobacco not only are implicated as causative factors of many head and neck cancers but their use can further compromise adequate nutrient intake. Thus, it is especially important that patients with head and neck cancer undergo pretreatment nutritional evaluation, appropriate nutritional support and monitoring during and close nutritional follow-up after treatment. The purpose of this article is to review the current literature supporting the benefit of nutritional support, patient assessment and nutritional repletion, and the advantages and disadvantages of various alimentation modalities.

Etiology and Types of Malnutrition

Formerly, the definition of malnutrition was based on population and individual patient anthropomorphic and laboratory values. Both the American Society of Parenteral and Enteral Nutrition and the Academy of Nutrition and Dietetics have recently developed standardized definitions for malnutrition based on a patient's degree of inflammation [6]. There are three major categories: simple starvation with no underlying inflammation; mild to moderate inflammation, which would include conditions such as cancer cachexia, pancreatitis, sarcopenic obesity and severe inflammation including trauma and sepsis. Because no single parameter defines adult malnutrition, the identification of two or more of the following six characteristics is recommended for diagnosis: 1) insufficient energy intake; 2) weight loss; 3) loss of muscle mass; 4) loss of subcutaneous fat; 5) localized or generalized fluid accumulation that may sometimes mask weight loss; and 6) diminished functional status as measured by handgrip strength [7].

Neoplasms of the head and neck can mechanically impede the intake of nourishment or cause trismus and odynophagia that limit oral intake [3]. The surgical and medical treatment regimens for head and neck cancer often result in side effects that cause anorexia and a decrease in oral intake. Surgical therapy can alter the anatomy such that chewing and swallowing can be temporarily or permanently dysfunctional [8]. Radiation therapy and chemotherapy commonly result in mucositis, dysgeusia, anosmia, xerostomia, trismus, nausea and vomiting [9]. Poor dentition may also contribute by increasing difficulty with mastication. Radiation-induced dental disease can further exacerbate this problem [10]. Alcohol and tobacco use, commonly seen in this patient group, add to the problem by providing "empty calories" devoid of essential nutrients and suppressing appetite. Patients who consume excessive amounts of alcohol have also been shown to have a much lower intake of fresh fruits and vegetables [7]. Diets low in essential vitamins and minerals are associated with increased risk of head and neck cancer.

Other factors that contribute to metabolic complications include tumor-induced metabolic dysfunction or cancer cachexia or immune and wound healing alterations. Downstream complications resulting from poor nutrition and its subsequent sequelae such as pneumonia, wound infections and sepsis can further increase inflammation and therefore increase nutritional demands. These demands often correspond to the time that per *os* nutrition is very limited or impossible, for example, the early postoperative period or during daily radiation treatments. The nutritional demands during this phase result in catabolism of stored glycogen (exhausted during the first 24 hrs.) and then corresponding loss of proteins in lean tissue. Fat is eventually mobilized to meet the nutritional needs: nutrition support must be addressed and initiated in the treatment plan to avoid such adverse outcomes.

Specific tumor-induced anorexia and accompanying metabolic dysfunction also contribute to malnutrition. Anorexia from cancer is thought to result from alterations in neurotransmitters, immunoregulatory hormones and possibly from learned food aversions [11]. Alterations in metabolism from solid tumors impact the body's metabolism as tumors only derive their energy from glucose. They are unable to use amino acids or fat to create energy. Tumorogenic and immune modulating factors (tumor necrosis factor [TNF], and interleukins IL-1, and IL-6) result in catabolism of muscle and tissue proteins, which are converted to glucose in the liver. Without normal immune responses, this available glucose helps drive cell replication by cancer cells [12]. Fat is also catabolized and elevated levels of plasma free fatty acids are thought to be secondary to hepatic neoketogenesis and are responsible for relative insulin insensitivity by normal body tissues. Insulin deficiency decreases normal tissue amino acid uptake and further fuels gluconeogenesis.

Impact of Malnutrition

The impact of malnutrition on patients is profound and directly impacts outcomes. Mick, et al. studied a group of patients with stage III & IV head and neck cancer treated with multiple modalities. The strongest independent predictor of survival was pretreatment weight loss [13]. Bertrand et al. showed that 7-10 days of preoperative nutrition resulted in a significant improvement in postoperative quality of life and led to a 10% decrease in postoperative infectious complications [14]. Van Bokhorst et al. showed that patients who have lost more than 10% of their ideal body weight are at increased risk of postoperative complications [15]. Malnourished patients are immuno-compromised with a particular decrease in cell-mediated immunity. Friedlander et al. found that the degree of malnutrition will correlate with the tumor burden and affect outcome; furthermore the immune suppression observed in malnourished patients is associated with the unimpeded tumor growth [16]. Malnourished and cachectic patients are also frequently unable to tolerate antineoplastic therapies that results in treatment delay and higher costs.

Nutritional Assessment

Because of the risks associated with malnutrition, it is important to be able to identify before treatment begins those head and neck cancer patients most at risk for malnutrition. Multiple assessment tools for malnutrition have been proposed. A complete history and physical exam is probably the most commonly used and best method of evaluating nutritional status. Components of the history that must be elicited include recent unintentional weight loss, loss of appetite and changes in endurance. Physical examination demonstrating sarcopenia or wasting is best demonstrated in the quadriceps femoris and the deltoid muscles. Cheilosis, stomatitis and dry scaling skin can be indicative of vitamin and other micronutrient deficiencies. Other parameters that can be used in nutrition assessment include anthropometric measurements (triceps skin fold, upper arm diameter).

Using weight as the sole marker of nutritional status is inadequate and even using traditional anthropometric measurements may not be sensitive to acute changes in nutrition [17]. Malnutrition has been defined as weight loss greater than 10% of ideal body weight that is associated with muscle wasting. The oldest method used to evaluate nutritional status is comparing body weight with usual or ideal body weight (IBW) using the Hamwi formula:

Men: ideal weight = 106 lb + 6 lb for every inch over 5 ft; Women: ideal weight = 100 lb + 5 lb for every inch over 5 ft.

Once the IBW is determined, the patient's weight loss as a percentage of IBW can then be determined as follows:

% Weight loss = (IBW – Admission weight / IBW) x 100.

More recently body mass index (BMI) may also be a useful tool to evaluate nutritional status. This index is calculated by weight in kilograms divided by the height in meters squared: BMI = weight (kg)/height (m^2). A BMI of ≤ 18.5 kg/m^2 is considered underweight, (table 1).

Several biochemical markers exist for testing nutritional status. Traditionally albumin, pre-albumin, and transferrin have been used to define nutritional depletion. However no single marker measures nutritional status accurately, (table 2). Albumin is the major protein produced by the liver and has a normal range of 3.5 g/dL to 4.5 g/dL. It functions as the major protein carrier and preserves intravascular oncotic pressure. Albumin has a half-life of

20 days and therefore poorly reflects acute changes in nutritional intake or status. Albumin however remains the defining factor in starvation and is the best serum marker to correlate with mortality rate in hospitalized patients [18].

Table 1. Malnutrition classification based on weight measurements

Index	Mild	Moderate	Severe	Appropriate weight
Weight loss (% IBW)	<10%	10-20%	>20%	>10%
BMI (kg/m2)	17–18.5	16– 16.9	< 16	18.5– 25

Body mass index (BMI).
Patient weight loss as a percentage (% IBW).

Table 2. Biomarkers utilized to assess the patient's nutritional status

Index	Mild	Moderate	Severe
Albumin (g/dL)	3.5-2.8	2.7-2.1	< 2.1
Transferrin (mg/dL)	200-151	150-100	< 100
Prealbumin (mg/dL)	15-10	9.9-5	< 5
Total Lymphocyte Count (per mm3)	1800-1500	1499-900	< 900

Transferrin is the major iron transport protein and has a circulating half-life of 8 days. It is synthesized by the liver and has a normal range of 200 mg/dL to 260 mg/dL. Iron metabolism and nutritional status affect its production, which may reduce its reliability as nutritional status marker [19]. Pre-albumin is synthesized by the liver and ranges from 15 mg/dL to 25 mg/dL. It too transports hormones and proteins I the serum and has a half-life of 2 to 3 days. Nutritional depletion is reflected by changes in pre-albumin sooner than by changes in albumin. Even though changes in nutrition intake can be seen as early as 7 days in the pre-albumin levels, fewer studies have validated its usefulness over albumin to predict outcome [20]. Several medical conditions such as renal insufficiency affect pre-albumin plasma levels.

Hemoglobin and hematocrit levels are measures of a continually changing protein compartment in the body that is adversely affected by many factors including both simple protein and caloric needs as well as vitamins and minerals (e.g., iron). Microcytic and macrocytic indices are well-known measures of folic acid and iron deficiencies that should be evaluated in every patient.

White blood cells are integrated into all phases of the response to injury, infection and inflammation and by their nature have relatively high metabolic needs. A total lymphocyte count below the range of 1200 to 1500/mm^3, lacking reasons for immunosuppression, is another indicator of malnutrition. Even other schema derived from many of the above parameters, such as creatinine-height index, prognostic nutritional index (PNI) and subjective global assessment (SGA) are used in identifying nutritionally deficient patients. SGA is unique in that it is validated tool used to assess weight history, physical assessment including muscle wasting, fat loss and edema as well as assessing gastrointestinal symptoms affecting nutritional intake

Regardless as to the method employed to assess, diagnose or monitor, once high-risk patients are identified, immediate intervention is mandated to result in a much improved outcome.

Treatment of Malnutrition

Patients with difficulty eating secondary to pain and anorexia are treated easily with simple medical interventions. Mucositis is common in patients receiving radiation therapy and chemotherapy. Treatment is generally with topical medications (analgesics, antifungals, coating agents and antihistamines) and gentle local care. Dental care can address pain of dental origin and frequent sips of water, synthetic saliva and pilocarpine can address problems of xerostomia. Patients who suffer from cancer-associated anorexia have shown good response to progestogens such as megestrol [21]. Other agents under investigation include ghrelin, thalidomide, anamorelin and eicosapentaenoic acid [22-25]. The dysgeusia experienced by patients who undergo radiation therapy and chemotherapy usually resolves within a year of treatment. Pain management is important as maximal medical therapy may not be able to completely alleviate the pain associated with these disorders.

Once a patient has been evaluated and his risk of malnutrition identified, nutritional counseling should be offered. Consulting a dietitian is appropriate whenever one identifies a patient currently malnourished or at risk of malnutrition. Their expertise is especially helpful when exploring the options for nutritional supplementation in patients with other medical problems. Patients who appear to be healthy should be counseled in regards to their diet and encouraged to eat a balanced diet with emphasis on high-protein, high-calorie foods. Expectations for future treatments and their influence on nutrition should be discussed. For patients with mild to moderate malnutrition who tolerate oral feeding, nutritional supplementation should be offered. Commercially available enteral formulas are constructed for complete nutritional supplementation meeting vitamin, protein and caloric established goals. However, home recipes using nutrient dense ingredients are equally suitable and may be less expensive. Liquid supplementation may not be necessary in patients who are able to chew and swallow effectively. They might be counseled to use whole milk instead of fat-free, real mayonnaise instead of dressing, butter, eggs, meats, legumes, ice cream and "instant breakfast" powders. These changes can significantly increase caloric intake with little change in actual volume. The patient should be encouraged to stop drinking alcohol and smoking tobacco too.

Methods of Nutritional Administration

Feeding tubes are placed into the gastrointestinal system effectively bypassing the most common areas of feeding difficulty for the patient with upper aerodigestive tract cancer. Dysphagia, odynophagia, and aspiration are usually not a concern once feeding is started through a nasogastric, gastrostomy or jejunostomy tubes. If the patient is cachectic or unable to satisfy his/her maintenance caloric needs by oral intake, he is a candidate for supplemental tube feeds. Gastrostomy tube placement before radiation therapy has been shown to prevent weight loss, treatment interruption, and dehydration [26]. In general, a nasogastric feeding tube should be used if expected length of use is less than 30 days. These tubes can irritate the nasal mucosa and may not be well tolerated. Tubes are made of either polyurethane (e.g., Ethox® *Ethox International, Buffalo, NY*, Compat® *Nestle HealthCare Nutrition Inc, Florham Park, NJ,* Dobbhof® *Covidien, Mansfield MA*) or silastic (such as NeoMed® *NeoMed Inc, Woodstock GA*) and offer many advantages over the rigid, larger polyvinyl chloride tubes (Levin® *One Medline Place, Mundelein Illinois)* or (Salem Sump® *Covidien, Mansfield MA)*. Due to their soft and small bore nature, these tubes decrease the incidence of nasal irritation and lower esophageal sphincter compromise thus decreasing the chance for reflux of gastric contents. The tip of the tube can be placed in the stomach or the small intestine. The pyloric sphincter acts as an additional barrier to refluxing feeds if patients are at high risk for complications of gastric feeding. Most authors feel that stomach feeds are more physiologic and are the first choice if aspiration risk is low.

If the patient is likely to require more than 30 days of tube feeds an enterocutaneous feeding tube is warranted. Enterocutaneous feeding tubes can be placed into the stomach or small bowel. They can be performed endoscopically, laparoscopically, open or under fluoroscopic guidance. Complications are rare with any of the applications, though morbidity is somewhat higher for open procedures. A prospective multi institution study of 172 head and neck cancer patients compared percutaneous endoscopically guided gastrostomy tube (PEG) insertion with radiologically inserted gastrostomy tubes (RIG) [27]. Within the series, mortality rates were noted at 1% for PEG and 3.9% for RIG. Major complication rates for PEG and RIG were 3.3% versus 15.6% respectively. There are case reports of cancer cells seeding the feeding tube site after endoscopic placement. Coletti et al. reported a case of tumor implantation into the abdominal wall after PEG placement in head and neck cancers patients [28]. He identified 41 case reports over the past two decades with roughly an incidence of up to 1%. This complication theoretically is avoided by "push" open or fluoroscopic procedures.

Placement of the tip of the feeding tube into the stomach is preferred regardless of which type of tube is used. The stomach acts as a reservoir, which allows for bolus feeds and allows for the administration of hypertonic feeds. If the patient has delayed emptying time or other gastric dysfunction as is often seen in the critically ill patient, a feeding tube placed into the small bowel may be more appropriate. Jejunal feeding was not shown to be superior when compared to gastrostomy tube in regard to risk of diarrhea, length of intensive care unit stay or decreased rate of pneumonia in critically ill patients [29, 30]. Bolus feeding is contraindicated when introducing enteral formulas into the small intestine. One study compared nasogastric tube placement with gastrostomy tube placement one day before surgery for either tonsillar or laryngeal squamous cell carcinoma. The authors found that patients spent a significantly shorter time in the hospital who received a gastrostomy tube [31]. Saunders et al. showed that patients tolerated gastrostomy tube placement long-term with high satisfaction levels [32].

Modalities of Nutritional Support

Patients who are judged at high risk and are unable to eat by mouth should be provided enteral feedings. There are two main routes of nutritional support: enteral and parenteral nutrition. Enteral nutrition is well tolerated and effective. There are a wide variety of enteral formulas available, (Table 3).

Osmolality affects the patient's ability to tolerate the formula [33]. High osmolality (> 1000 mOsm/kg) refers to a hypertonic formula that should be infused into the stomach to take advantage of the dilutional effects of the gastric secretion to prevent diarrhea [34]. Most enteral formulas are well tolerated with osmolalites ranging from 300 to700 mOsm/kg. The osmolality of the enteral formulas is determined by the most abundant nutrient and whether the formula is polymeric or predigested. The smaller molecules typically translate to a higher solute load [34]. Most enteral feeding formulas contain 1 kcal/mL, and are typically iso-osmolar. Although some enteral feeding formulas have 2 kcal/mL and are appropriate for patients who have increased caloric needs or volume constraints. In general, enteral feeding formulas can be separated into polymeric, monomeric and disease-specific formulations. Polymeric contain carbohydrate polymers, complete proteins and triglycerides. They can be used safely in the vast majority of patients. These formulas can be instilled in the stomach or small intestine. Monomeric formulations are essentially the predigested products of the polymeric formula. As such it contains carbohydrates in the form of oligosaccharides or maltodextrin, protein in the form of short peptide chains or free amino acids and lipids as a mixture of short and long-chain triglycerides. Monomeric formulations are considered more appropriate for patients with poor absorption or other digestion dysfunction. There have been no studies to clearly confirm the benefit of their use. Disease-specific formulas are made specific to a patient's disease state. Enteral feeding formulas rich in *Arginine*, *glutamine* and *Omega-3 fatty acids* are thought to alter immune function [35-37]. This leads to their increased use for cancer patients. Although an analysis of relevant studies failed to show any survival benefit in cancer patients, a decrease in post-operative infection rates has been reported [38]. Formulas with Eicosapentaenoic acid (EPA) / Dexahexanoic acid (DHA) have also been shown to be helpful in patients with significant cancer cachexia [39, 40].

Current recommendations for enteral feeding administration are that feedings should be started with full-strength formula, initiated and steadily increased to goal when there is no formula intolerance and to achieve full nutrient intake as soon as possible [34, 41, 42]. Conservative initiation and advancement rates are reserved for patients who have not been fed for some time and are receiving high-osmolality or calorie dense formula [41]. Two types of enteral feeding protocols have been categorized: bolus feeding and continuous infusion. Bolus feedings are used primarily in patients who have nasogastric or gastrostomy feeding tubes. Continuous infusion is indicated when the patient has nasojejunal, gastojejunal or jejunal feeding tubes. Caloric needs are best estimated at 25-35 kcal/kg/day for maintenance and to support nutritional repletion. Contrary to widespread opinion, evidence from clinical studies and animal experiments suggests that initiating early enteral feedings is advantageous and specifically associated with an improvement in wound healing [43].

Table 3. Selected commercially available enteral formulas

Product	Manufacture	Kcal/ml	Protein %	Carbohydrate%	Fat %	Osmolarity mOsm/kg
Nutren 1.0	Nestlé Nutrition (Highland Park, MI)	1	16%	51%	33%	315
Nutren 2.0	Nestlé Nutrition (Highland Park, MI)	2	16%	39%	45%	746
Vivonex T.E.N.	Nestlé Nutrition (Highland Park, MI)	1	15%	82%	3%	630
Isosource HN	Sandoz Inc (East Hanover, NJ)	1.2	18%	53%	29%	490
Fibersource HN	Sandoz Inc (East Hanover, NJ)	1.2	18%	53%	29%	490
Jevity 1 Cal	Abbott Nutrition (Columbus, OH)	1.06	17%	54%	29%	300
Boost	Nestlé Nutrition (Highland Park, MI)	1	17%	68%	15%	625
Ensure Plus	Abbott Nutrition (Columbus, OH)	1.5	15%	56%	15%	470
Osmolite 1.2 Cal	Abbott Nutrition (Columbus, OH)	1.2	19%	53%	29%	360

Parenteral nutrition is the feeding option of "last resort" and should be employed only when enteral feeding is not possible or is contraindicated. Total Parenteral Nutrition (TPN) can be valuable when treating severely malnourished patients who need immediate metabolic treatment or who have lost small bowel function. This intervention is much more expensive, requires a central line and is associated with significant complications [44]. The formula is a hypertonic mixture of amino acids, dextrose, fat emulsions, vitamins, trace elements and electrolytes. Insulin can be added to the formula to treat hyperglycemia which may occur with infusions of hypertonic dextrose. This allows for automatic titration of the insulin to the amount of formula being administered. TPN requires daily electrolyte monitoring and composition adjustment. Complications include line-related problems, infection, sepsis and metabolic complications [45, 46]. Patients are typically weaned off TPN before surgery to avoid inadvertent hyper/hypoglycemia [47].

Studies have shown improvement in postoperative morbidity in malnourished patients receiving TPN when they are fed for 7-10 days preoperatively [48]. When compared with enteral nutrition, TPN provides no added benefit over enteral feeds [49].

Looking to the Future

Dietary causes for cancers are being demonstrated in certain populations (oral cancer with betel nuts, esophageal cancer with smoked foods) and to prevent such cancers by altering the diet is one of the most exciting new oncologic concepts. Some authors have investigated food-related substances in an effort to identify which foods might offer a protective value against head and neck cancer. Low serum levels of vitamin A or beta-carotene have been associated with cancer of the head and neck and gastric cancer [50]. Schantz, et al. showed an increased risk of head and neck cancer in patients who ate foods deficient in cryptoxanthin, lycopene and Vitamins C and E and they postulated that these substances might act as free radical scavengers and thus "protect" DNA from mutation [51]. Recently, studies looking at N-3 polyunsaturated fatty acids derived from fish oils have shown some positive effects in patients who are immunocompromised [52, 53]. This resulted in development of special enteral formulas that contain Arginine, dietary nucleotides and N-3 fatty acids. Prospective studies have shown improvement in postoperative infection rates in head and neck cancer patients when immunoenhanced enteral formulas are used [54]. A meta-analysis of these studies however showed no added benefit when compared with the use of conventional enteral feeds [55].

Conclusion

Comprehensive care of head and neck cancer patients must include a thorough evaluation of their nutritional status prior to initiating cancer treatment and frequent re-evaluation during and after therapy. Once a patient has been identified as being malnourished they should be assessed for their ability to take food by mouth and a coordinated nutritional treatment plan must be developed. Appropriate supplementation should be provided if necessary. Enteral feeding is very successful in bypassing disease states of the upper aerodigestive system and results in improvement in treatment tolerance, post-treatment morbidity, long-term quality of life and decreased mortality. Alternative medical interventions may also be effective as adjuvant therapies.

References

[37] Van Bokhorst DS, van Leeuwen PA, Kuik DJ, Klop WM, Sauerwein HP, Snow GB, Quak JJ. The impact of nutritional status on the prognoses of patients with advanced head and neck cancer. *Cancer* 86:519–527, 1999.

[38] Eley KA, Shah R, Bond SE, Watt-Smith SR. A review of post-operative feeding in patients undergoing resection and reconstruction for oral malignancy and presentation of a pre-operative scoring system. *Br J Oral Maxillofac Surg* 50:601-605, 2012.

[39] O'Neill J, Shaha A. Nutrition Management of Patients with Malignancies of the Head and Neck. *Surg Clin N Am* 91:631–639, 2011.

[40] Boyle JO, Gumus ZH, Choksi VL, Bocker JM, Zhou XK, Yantiss RK, Hughes DB, Du B, Judson BL, Subbaramaiah K, Dannenberg AJ. Effects of cigarette smoke on the human oral mucosal transcriptome. *Cancer Prev Res* 3:266–278, 2010.

[41] Ravasco P, Monteiro-Grillo I, Vidal PM, Camilo ME. Nutritional deterioration in cancer: The role of disease and diet. *Clin Oncol* (R Coll Radiol) 15:443-450, 2003.

[42] White JV, Guenter P, Jensen G Malone A, Schofield M; Academy Malnutrition Work Group; A.S.P.E.N. Malnutrition Task Force; A.S.P.E.N. Board of Directors. Consensus statement: Academy of Nutrition and Dietetics and American Society of Parenteral and Enteral Nutrition: Characteristics recommended for the identification and documentation of adult malnutrition (undernutrition). *JPEN J Parenter Enteral Nutr* 36:275-283, 2012.

[43] Ross LJ, Wilson M, Banks M, Rezannah F, Daglish M. Prevalence of malnutrition and nutritional risk factors in patients undergoing alcohol and drug treatment. *Nutrition* 28:738-743, 2012.

[44] Beeken L, Calman F. A return to ''normal eating'' after curative treatment for oral cancer. What are the long-term prospects? *Eur J Cancer B Oral Oncol.* 30:387–392, 1994.

[45] Beaver MES, Matheny KE, Roberts DB, Myers JN. Predictors of weight loss during radiation therapy. *Otolaryngol Head Neck Surg* 125:645–658, 2001.

[46] Badwal R.S., Bennett J. Nutritional considerations in the surgical patient. *Dent Clin N Am* 47:373–393, 2003.

[47] Monteleone P. New frontiers in endocrinology of eating disorders. *Curr Top Behav Neurosci* 6:189-208, 2011.

[48] George J, Cannon T, Lai V, Richey L, Zanation A, Hayes DN, Shores C, Guttridge D, Couch M. Cancer cachexia syndrome in head and neck cancer patients: Part II. Pathophysiology. *Head Neck* 29:497-507, 2007.

[49] Mick R, Vokes EE, Weichselbaum RR, Panje WR. Prognostic factors in advanced head and neck cancer patients undergoing multimodality therapy. *Otolaryngol Head Neck Surg* 105:62-73, 1991.

[50] Bertrand PC, Piquet MA, Bordier I, Monnier P, Roulet M. Preoperative nutritional support at home in head and neck cancer patients: from nutritional benefits to the prevention of the alcohol withdrawal syndrome. *Curr Opin Clin Nutr Metab Care* 5:435-440, 2002.

[51] Van Bokhorst-de van der Schueren MA, van Leeuwen PA, Sauerwein HP, Kuik DJ, Snow GB, Quak JJ. Assessment of malnutrition parameters in head and neck cancer and their relation to postoperative complications. *Head Neck* 5:419-425, 1997.

[52] Friedlander A, TajimaT, Kawakami K, Wang M, Tomlinson J. The Relationship between Measures of Nutritional Status and Masticatory Function in Untreated Patients with Head and Neck Cancer. *J Oral Maxillofac Surg* 66:85-92, 2008.

[53] Carney DE, Meguid MM. Current concepts in nutritional assessment. Arch Surg 137:42–44, 2002.

[54] Gibbs J, Cull W, Henderson W, Daley J, Hur K, Khuri SF. Preoperative serum albumin level as a predictor of operative mortality and morbidity. *Arch Surg* 134:36–42, 1999.

[55] Fang J, Chirag D, Dym H. Nutritional Aspects of Care. *Oral Maxillofacial Surg Clin N Am* 18: 115–130, 2006.

[56] Mittman N, Avram MM, Oo KK, Chattopadhyay J. Serum prealbumin predicts survival in hemodialysis and peritoneal dialysis: 10 years of prospective observation. *Am J Kidney Dis* 38:1358-1364, 2001.

[57] Berenstein EG, Ortiz Z. Megestrol acetate for the treatment of anorexia-cachexia syndrome. *Cochrane Database Syst Rev* 18:CD004310, 2005.

[58] Yennurajalingam S, Willey JS, Palmer JL, Allo J, Fabbro ED, Cohen EN, Tin S, Reuben JM, Bruera E. The Role of Thalidomide and Placebo

for the Treatment of Cancer-Related Anorexia-Cachexia Symptoms: Results of a Double-Blind Placebo-Controlled Randomized Study. *J Palliat Med* 10: 1059-1064, 2012.

[59] Fujitsuka N, Asakawa A, Amitani H, Hattori T, Inui A. Efficacy of ghrelin in cancer cachexia: clinical trials and a novel treatment by rikkunshito. *Crit Rev Oncog* 17:277-284, 2012.

[60] Garcia JM, Friend J, Allen S. Therapeutic potential of anamorelin, a novel, oral ghrelin mimetic, in patients with cancer-related cachexia: a multicenter, randomized, double-blind, crossover, pilot study. *Support Care Cancer* 21: 129-137, 2013.

[61] Murphy RA, Yeung E, Mazurak VC, Mourtzakis M. Influence of eicosapentaenoic acid supplementation on lean body mass in cancer cachexia. *Br J Cancer* 105:1469-1473, 2011.

[62] Beaver ME, Matheny KE, Roberts DB. Predictors of weight loss during radiation therapy. *Otolaryngol Head Neck Surg* 125: 645–648, 2001.

[63] Grant D, Bradley P, Pothier D. Complications following gastrostomy tube insertion in patients with head and neck cancer: a prospective multi-institution study, systematic review and meta-analysis. *Clin Otolaryngol* 34:103-112, 2009.

[64] Coletti D, Genuit T, Ord R, Engroff S. Metastasis to the Percutaneous Endoscopic Gastrostomy Site in the Patient with Head and Neck Cancer: A Case Report and Review of the Literature. *J Oral Maxillofac Surg* 64:1149-1157, 2006.

[65] Ho KM, Dobb GJ, Webb SA. A comparison of early gastric and post-pyloric feeding in critically ill patients: a meta-analysis. *Intensive Care Med* 32:639-649, 2006.

[66] Drover JW. Gastric versus postpyloric feeding. *Gastrointest Endosc Clin N Am* 17:765-775, 2007.

[67] Gibson S, Wenig BL. Percutaneous endoscopic gastrostomy in the management of head and neck carcinoma. *Laryngoscope* 102:977-980, 1992.

[68] Saunders JR, Brown MS, Hirata RM, Jaques DA. Percutaneous endoscopic gastrostomy in patients with head and neck malignancies. *Am J Surg* 162:381-383, 1991.

[69] Stuart S, Stuart M, Unger LD. Enteral and parenteral nutrition support. In: Morrison G, Hark L, editors. Medical nutrition and disease. *Cambridge (MA) Blackwell Science,* 1996, pp. 339–352.

[70] Marino PL. *Enteral nutrition*. In: Zinner SR. The ICU book. 3rd Edition Baltimore (MD): Williams & Wilkins, 2007, pp. 891–893.

[71] Shang HF, Wang YY, Lai YN, Chiu WC, Yeh SL. Effects of arginine supplementation on mucosal immunity in rats with septic peritonitis. *Clin Nutr* 23:561-569, 2004.

[72] Lai YN, Yeh SL, Lin MT, Shang HF, Yeh CL, Chen WJ. Glutamine supplementation enhances mucosal immunity in rats with Gut-Derived sepsis. *Nutrition* 20:286-291, 2004.

[73] Senkal M, Kemen M, Homann HH, Eickhoff U, Baier J, Zumtobel V. Modulation of postoperative immune response by enteral nutrition with a diet enriched with arginine, RNA, and omega-3 fatty acids in patients with upper gastrointestinal cancer. *Eur J Surg* 161:115-122, 1995.

[74] Stableforth WD, Thomas S, Lewis SJ. A systematic review of the role of immunonutrition in patients undergoing surgery for head and neck cancer. *Int J Oral Maxillofac Surg* 38:103-110, 2009.

[75] Couch M, Lai V, Cannon T, Guttridge D, Zanation A, George J, Hayes DN, Zeisel S, Shores C. Cancer cachexia syndrome in head and neck cancer patients: part I. Diagnosis, impact on quality of life and survival, and treatment. *Head Neck* 29:401-411, 2007.

[76] Braga M, Gianotti L, Nespoli L, Radaelli G, Di Carlo V. Nutritional approach in the malnourished surgical patient: A prospective randomized study. *Arch Surg* 137:174-180, 2002.

[77] Margenthaler JA, Herrmann VM. Doherty GM, Lowney JK, Mason JE. *The Washington manual of surgery.* 3rd edition. Philadelphia (PA). Lippincott, Williams & Wilkins, 2002, pp. 9–26.

[78] Rees RG, Keohane PP, Grimble GK, Frost PG, Attrill H, Silk DB. Elemental diet administered nasogastrically without starter regimens to patients with inflammatory bowel disease. *JPEN J Parenter Enteral Nutr* 10:258–262, 1986.

[79] Lewis SJ, Egger M, Sylvester PA, Thomas S: Early enteral feeding versus "nil by mouth" after gastrointestinal surgery: systemic review and meta-analysis of controlled trials. *BMJ* 323: 1-5, 2001.

[80] Dudrick SJ, Pimiento JM. Parenteral nutrition and nutritional support of surgical patients: reflections, controversies, and challenges. *Surg Clin North Am* 91:675-692, 2011.

[81] Sena MJ, Utter GH, Cuschieri J, Maier RV, Tompkins RG, Harbrecht BG, Moore EE, O'Keefe GE. Early supplemental parenteral nutrition is associated with increased infectious complications in critically ill trauma patients. *J Am Coll Surg* 207:459-567, 2008.

[82] Simpson F, Doig GS. Parenteral vs. enteral nutrition in the critically ill patient: a meta-analysis of trials using the intention to treat principle. *Intensive Care Med* 31:12-23, 2005.

[83] Kumar PR, Crotty P, Raman M. Hyperglycemia in hospitalized patients receiving parental nutrition is associated with increased morbidity and mortality: a review. *Gastroenterol Res Pract* 10: 1155-1162, 2011.

[84] Heyland DK, Montalvo M, MacDonald S, Keefe L, Su XY, Drover JW. Total parenteral nutrition in the surgical patient: a meta-analysis. *Can J Surg* 44:102-111, 2001.

[85] Gramlich L, Kichian K, Pinilla J, Rodych NJ, Dhaliwal R, Heyland DK. Does enteral nutrition compared to parenteral nutrition result in better outcomes in critically ill adult patients? A systematic review of the literature. *Nutrition* 20:843-848, 2004.

[86] Abnet CC, Qiao YL, Dawsey SM, Buckman DW, Yang CS, Blot WJ, Dong ZW, Taylor PR, Mark SD. Prospective study of serum retinol, beta-carotene, beta-cryptoxanthin, and lutein/zeaxanthin and esophageal and gastric cancers in China. *Cancer Causes Control* 14:645-655, 2003.

[87] Schantz SP, Zhang ZF, Spitz MS, Sun M, Hsu TC. Genetic susceptibility to head and neck cancer: interaction between nutrition and mutagen sensitivity. *Laryngoscope* 107:765-781, 1997.

[88] Liang B, Wang S, Ye YJ, Yang XD, Wang YL, Qu J, Xie QW, Yin MJ. Impact of postoperative omega-3 fatty acid-supplemented parenteral nutrition on clinical outcomes and immunomodulations in colorectal cancer patients. *World J Gastroenterol* 14:2434-2439, 2008.

[89] Heller AR, Rössler S, Litz RJ, Stehr SN, Heller SC, Koch R, Koch T. Omega-3 fatty acids improve the diagnosis-related clinical outcome. *Crit Care Med* 34:972-979, 2006.

[90] Casas-Rodera P, Gómez-Candela C, Benítez S, Mateo R, Armero M, Castillo R, Culebras JM. Immunoenhanced enteral nutrition formulas in head and neck cancer surgery: a prospective, randomized clinical trial. *Nutr Hosp* 23:105-110, 2008.

[91] Wilhelm SM, Kale-Pradhan PB. Combination of arginine and omega-3 fatty acids enteral nutrition in critically ill and surgical patients: a meta-analysis. *Expert Rev Clin Pharmacol* 3:459-469, 2010.

In: Parenteral Nutrition
Editor: Shana Lelio

ISBN: 978-1-63321-112-4

Chapter 3

Nutrition Support Teams and the Role of Registered Dietitians

Conxita Mestres Miralles*
Faculty of Heath Sciences Blanquerna, University Ramon Llull, Barcelona, Spain

Abstract

Nutritional counseling by RD has demonstrated that improves the quality of life through nutrient intake in hospitalized patients. In the last decades the role of registered dietitians (RD) has evolved including new responsibilities, activities and areas of work.

Between these, it is the integration of RD in nutrition support teams, with other professionals as physicians, pharmacists and nurses. One of the major roles of these teams is improving the safety and effectiveness of Parenteral Nutrition, therefore RD knowledge is of great interest in the management of critically ill patients. RD attends daily rounds, manage complex nutrition therapies and participate in policy and protocol development, perform research, feedback and education to other professionals. Other activities of RD is to document in the patient`s progress notes recommendations to the attending physician and bring information about: anthropometrics, fluid status, amount of nutrition received and estimated nutrition needs.

* Pharm Dr., Associate Professor. Faculty of Heath Sciences Blanquerna. University Ramon Llull. , Padilla 326. 08025 Barcelona (Spain), concepciomm@blanquerna.url.edu.

There are some settings, where RD has been granted privileges for order writing. Thus leading to greater assurance that an intervention will occur, improving nutritional status, better glycemic, caloric and electrolytic control as well as reduction in inappropriate parenteral nutritional use and cost savings.

Therefore, RD has to continue to integrate and expand their role in the management of parenteral nutrition, in Intensive Care Units (UCI) and in less critical patients who are taking artificial nutrition.

Introduction

It is known that malnutrition in hospitals is a great problem affecting 20-60% of the patients, increasing the length of hospital stay, comorbility, mortality and decreasing quality of life. [1, 2] This is translated to important costs for the healthcare systems, a study in the United Kingdom in 2005 showed that the cost of disease-related to malnutrition where of £ 7.4 billion [3].

A meeting held in November 2012, organized by the European Heath Management Association (EHMA) and the Heath Care Federation (HOPE) brought together European experts in Nutrition to identify key barriers to solve this problem and to look at potential strategies to ensure good nutrition [4]. At the end of the meeting some priorities were established that included between others:

- Introduction of Nutrition Support Teams with clear definition and responsibilities
- Creation of integrative financing process with diagnosis related group (DRG)

Different causes and barriers have been identified in the prevention and management of under-nutrition in health care institutions, such as:

- Lack of time, staff shortage and pour interdisciplinary collaboration.
- Inadequate nutritional assessment and support
- Inadequate medical knowledge and practice in the field of nutrition
- Erroneous idea that it has not an important impact in patient outcome.
- Limited involvement and interest of hospital managers
- Financial resources and reimbursement systems are problematic.

Studies published have shown that nutrition interventions have positive outcomes and the usefulness of dietitian counseling in health care settings. A National Confidential Enquiry conducted in England, on Patients Outcomes and Death report showed that metabolic complications occurred in 40-49% of the patients could have been avoided and that there were deficiencies in the assessment and monitoring of patients on PN in 54% of cases [5].

Therefore, in this line, the emergence and expansion of Nutrition Support Teams has been a great improvement.

Nutrition Support Teams

In specialized nutrition therapy (parenteral and enteral nutrition), an interdisciplinary approach is essential due to its risks and complexity (glucose, electrolyte and fluid imbalances, infections, acid-base alterations). In the 80's we saw the beginning of the creation of nutrition support teams in the hospitals. The structure of these teams depends on the institution particularities, needs and budgets, the professionals involved are physicians, pharmacists, nurses and dietitians, and have broad functions: [6, 7]

- Patient assessment: Clinical record, survey about previous nutritional habits, changes in corporal weight. Gravimetric and anthropometric measurements. Nutritional diagnostic. Establish nutritional needs: macro and micronutritents in relation to the nutritional status of the patient.
- Indication and withdrawn criteria assessment.
- Preparing and adapting the PN composition or selecting the commercially available.
- Monitoring and controlling of sterility, compatibility and stability of the PN.
- Advise wards on hygiene and compatibility aspects, how PN should be administered (e.g., accesses, tubes, pumps)
- Daily following of the patient constants (temperature, glycemia, diuresis, and other losses) related to the nutrition.
- Analytical control (creatinin, urea, hepatic enzymes, bilirrubin, lipids, total proteins, albumin, electrolytes, ferritin, iron, transferring ,phosphorous, magnesium, calcium, chloride, linocuts, and others)

- Management of mechanic, metabolic, electrolytic and hepatic complications related to the PN.
- Include in the clinical record all the information related to the PN.
- Participation in the Nutrition Committee.
- Establish guidelines and protocols related to the parenteral nutrition
- Evaluation of PN costs aspects
- Formative activities

Based on a survey conducted by the American Society for Parenteral and Enteral Nutrition (A.S.P.E.N), published in 2010, 42% of hospitals in the USA had a nutrition support team. But, the percentage decreased to only 28% for medium-small hospitals [8]. There is some lack of information in Europe; however, a survey conducted in England published in 2011 from 196 hospitals, showed that only 1.9% of the Intensive Care Units (ICU) had a team and 4.7% did not have a dietitian [9]. Another European survey found that teams were present at 2.83% of 2221 German hospitals, 7.92% of 278 Austrian hospitals and 2.45% of 572 Swiss hospitals. [10].

Therefore, there still yet a long task to do in order to expand the implementation of these teams, in hospitals, home care and nursing homes. Moreover, Parenteral Nutrition (PN) is also increasingly administered at home. Complication rates seem to be low [11] and is especially suitable for patients with short bowel syndrome due to Crohn's disease or other forms of intestinal failure, after intestinal ischemia, tumors, radioenteritis, and severe colonic disorders. In this setting, nutrition team, to the functions listed before, it should be added, to give information, clarification and consent to patients and relatives.

Another point to improve nutrition that can be accomplished by Nutrition Support Teams is to do measurements and introduce indicators in order to improve the quality of nutrition support. Goals can be fixed and if not meet, review practices and makes the necessary changes. Some of these could be [6, 12]:

- Percentage of patients for whom the nutrition support is indicated according to predefined standards (standards established by the institution or by national or international nutrition societies)
- Incidence of complications as:
  - Patients (%) with triglycerides > 400 mg/dl
  - Patients (%) with glycemia > 400 mg/dl

    - Hepatic alterations due to NP
- Percentage of valued patients
- Percentage of patients with daily following of constants.
- Percentage of patients whose nutritional support deviates from the prescribed treatment
- Percentage of patients with PN > 7 days

The involvement of dietitians in the management of parenteral nutrition (PN), has been increasing since the 1970s, however it is relatively recent compared with the other professionals, whose roles are better established (Table 1)

Table 1. Potential roles of professionals in the management of parenteral nutrition

• Physicians:
– Patient screening and assessment.
– Implementation of nutrition
– Patient monitoring
– Termination of therapy
• Pharmacists:
– Compound parenteral nutrition
– Control stability, compatibility and sterility
– Direct care patient
– Education of other health care professionals
– Research
• Nurses:
– Patient care
– Recognize side effects and complications
– Education of caregivers and patients
– Research

The role of registered dietitian (RD) has emerged as a specialty practice within professional dietetics with privileges to perform advanced clinical care. Clinical privileges are defined as "authorization granted by the appropriate authority to a practitioner to provide specific care, treatment, and services in an organization within well-defined limits, based on the following factors, as applicable: license, education, training, experience, competence, heath status and, judgment". [13]

Roles of Registered Dietitians in the Management of Parenteral Nutrition in Nutrition Support Teams

RD play or can play different roles alone or in cooperation with the other members of the nutrition support team, as:

Nutritional screening and assessment. This is a traditional role played by dietitians that have a specific education and training in this the area. Dietitian's competencies include confirming that PN is appropriate and assess patient's nutritional requirements in relation to their clinical status, making an evaluation between illness and malnutrition and make PN recommendations. Some authors have demonstrated that average time to reach nutritional requirements was improved with the following of dietitian recommendations [14].

Develop nutrition plans. After assessing the needs of the patient, in collaboration with pharmacists, nurses and physicians, they establish an individualized nutrition plan.

Attending daily rounds, dietitians can assess the state of patients and adjust nutritional requirements in function of their evolution and managing complex PN. The presence of dietitians has been found to increase the adherence to guidelines in the nutritional management of UCI patients [15]

They also participate in *developing transitional feeding care plan* or *termination of nutrition support,* assessing patient's tolerance and intake of oral/enteral nutrition.

As member of the interdisciplinary team, dietitians participate in the *development of parenteral nutrition protocols and guidelines.* As well as *educating* other healthcare professionals, students, patients and caregivers and *perform nutrition-related research.* [3]

Registered Dietitian Order Writing Privileges

As we have seen so far, even though, dietitians have important roles in the nutritional support team, therapeutic diets, due to regulatory standards, have been prescribed by the practitioner/s responsible of the patient.

A.S.P.E.N and the American Dietetic Association (ADA) have established standards of practice and standards of professional performance for RD in nutritional support [16]. In this document there are descriptions of advanced practices in nutrition support that include processes to empower RD with privileges for nutrition order writing in long-term and acute-care hospitals.

In February 2013 [17] Centers for Medicare and Medicaid Services (CMS) have proposed a rule change that would permit registered dietitians (who have been granted privileges by their hospital), to order patient diets independently of physicians and order laboratory tests to monitor the effectiveness of dietary plans and orders. The change is expected to take effect soon, when it would be finalized by CMS.

The American Dietetic Association estates the importance of this rule in order to:

- Save hospital resources, as physicians will have more time to devote to their patients
- RD is the best qualified to ass's patient's nutritional status and perform the designing of diets and nutritional plans in collaboration with the nutrition support team.

Between 2006 and 2007 a study was conducted [18] in order to compare PN use before RD order-writing privileges and after granting them. Results showed that PN decreased from 1080 to 885, even though the number of hospital admissions in this period had increased, inappropriate PN also decreased from 45% to 27%. Inappropriate PN use included patients with poor oral intake, pancreatitis, intractable nausea and vomiting and mucositits. No significant differences were found in the hospital length of stay, intensive care admissions or other complications.

Conclusion

The awareness of the prevalence and importance of under-nutrition in patients in health care settings has been increasing in the last decades. The great improvement that can be accomplished in this field by Nutrition Support Teams has been recognized. The collaboration between physicians, nurses, pharmacists and dietitians has shown to be the better way to affront thins challenge. However, there is a long way to make, especially due to the shortage of financial founds in health care and that persists a lack of understanding of the importance of nutrition support in the outcomes of patients.

In the area of PN, is where the Nutrition Support Teams emerged and where more has been improved. The role of dietitians in these Teams has more importance day to day, and it seems that is expanding, as has been seen in some experiences and perspectives about increasing their privileges, even to order-writing.

All this implies that RD and the other professionals involved, in the near future, should need a high and specialized formation and knowledge in PN and all the implications in the outcome and benefits of the patients.

References

[1] Rüfenacht U, Rühlin M, Wegmann M, Imoberdorf R, Ballmer P. Nutritional counseling improves quality of life and nutrient intake in undernourished patients. *Nutrition*.2010, 26:53-60

[2] Sorensen J, Kondrup J, Prokopowicz J, Schiesser M, Krahenbuhl L, Meier R et al. EuroOOPS: an international, multicentre study to implement nutritional risk screening and evaluate clinical outcome. *Clin Nutr.* 2008:27(3)340-7

[3] National Confidential Enquiry into Patients Outcome and Death (NCEPOD) report (2010). Parenteral nutrition: a mixed bag 2010. Parenteral Nutrition toolkit. *http://www.ncepod.org.uk/2010pn.htm*

[4] Under-Nutrition. Removing barriers to efficient patient nutrition within both the hospital and home-care setting. 2012 *http://www.hope.be/05eventsandpublications/docpublications/93_nutrition/93_HOPE-EHMA_Under-nutrition_May_2013pdf.pdf*

[5] DeLegge MH, Kelley AT. State of Nutrition Support Teams. *Nutr. Clin. Practice*. 2013,28:691-7.

[6] López Martin C, Abilés J, Garrido Siles M, Faus Felipe V. *Impact of the creations of a nutritional support team on the quality, safety and effectiveness of total parenteral nutrition.* Nutrición Hospitalaria, 2012, 27:871-8

[7] Bischhoff SC, Kester L, Meier R, Radziwill R, Schwab D, Thul P, Working group for developing the guidelines for parenteral nutrition of The German Association for Nutritional Medicine. Organization, regulations, preparation and logistics of parenteral nutrition in hospitals

and homes; the role of nutrition support team- Guidelines on Parenteral Nutrition.Chapter 8, *GMS Ger Med Sci* 2009:7,Doc 20.

[8] ASPEN Practice Management Task Force, DeLegge M, Wooley J, Guenter P, Wright S, Brill J, Andris D, Wagner P, Filibeck D. A.S.P.E.N. Board of Directors. The Status of Nutrition Support Teams and Update of Current Models for Providing Nutrition Support Therapy to Patients. *Nutr. Clin. Pract.* 2010,25 (1):76-84

[9] Sharifi MN, Walton A, Chakrabarty G, Rahman T, Neild P, Poullis A. Nutrition support in intensive care units in England: a snapshot of present practice. *British J Nutr.* 2011, 106: 1240-4.

[10] Shang E, Hasenberg B, Schlegel B, Sterchi AB, Schindler K, Druml W, Koletzko B, Meier R. An European survey of structure and organization of nutrition support teams in Germany, Austria and Switzerland. *Clin. Nutr.* 2005,24:1005-13.

[11] Howard L, Ashley C. Management of complications in patients receiving home parenteral nutrition. *Gastroenterology*.2003:124. 161-61.

[12] Braunschweig CL, Raizman DJ, Kovacevich, Keresten-Smith JK. Impact of the clinical nutritionist on tube feeding administration, *J. Am. Diet. Assoc.* 1998,88:664-86

[13] Joint Commission on Accreditation of Healthcare Organizations. 2006. Hospital Accreditation Standards. *Joint Commission Resources.* Inc. Oak Book.IL.,2006

[14] Schneider P. Nutrition Support Teams: An Evidence-Based Practice. *Nutr.Clin.Practice*. 2006.21:62-7

[15] Heyland D, Heyland R, Cahill N et al. Crating a culture of clinical excellence in critical care nutrition. *J Parenter.Enteral Nutr.*2010,34:707-15.

[16] A.S.P.E.N Board of Directors and ADA Quality Management Committee. American Society for Parenteral and Enteral Nutrition (A.S.P.E.N) and American Dietetic Association (ADA): Standards of Practice and Standards of Professional Performance for Registered Dietitians (Generalist, Specialty, and Advanced) in Nutrition Support. *Nutr. Clin.Pract.*2007,22: 558-86.

[17] CMS Proposed Rule Related to Therapeutic Diet Orders. Academy of Nutrition and Dietetics. *http://www.eatright.org/HealthProfessionals/ content.aspx?id=6442474904;http://www.eatright.org/dietorders/ Accessed March 10th 2014.*

[18] Peterson SJ, Chen Y, Sullivan CA, Kinnare K, Tupesis NC, Patel GP, Spwa DC, Lateef O. Assessing the Influence of Registered Dietitian Order-Writing Privileges on Parenteral Nutrition Use. *J.Am.Diet.Assoc.*2010, 110:1703-11.

In: Parenteral Nutrition
Editor: Shana Lelio

ISBN: 978-1-63321-112-4

Chapter 4

Parenteral Nutrition Associated Liver Disease: A Current Review Focused on the Infant

A. R. Hall, C. J. Arnold, G. A. Zello and G. G. Miller
Department of Surgery and College of Pharmacy and Nutrition,
University of Saskatchewan, Saskatoon, Canada

Abstract

Parenteral nutrition associated liver disease (PNALD) is one of the most common complications of neonatal parenteral nutrition, yet much of its pathogenesis and treatment remains a mystery. In infants, this disease encompasses a spectrum of hepatobiliary changes including both cholestasis and fibrosis; but not generally steatosis. The earliest stage is often signaled by a serum direct bilirubin of >2mg/dL (>34μmol/L) while dependent on parenteral nutrition (PN). If the child remains reliant on PN, the cholestasis may progress to portal hypertension, cirrhosis, and eventually end-stage liver disease. Although a definitive treatment for PNALD does not exist, considerable research on the topic has been conducted, thus a review of the literature is the first step to better understand this illness.

In the following chapter we outline the history and incidence of this disease, beginning with the first reporting in the early 1970s to its current presence in modern neonatal intensive care units. We then explore the multiple factors believed to contribute to PNALD, including immature neonatal handling of bile (especially in those born premature) and a lack of enteral stimulation seen in those infants solely dependent on PN. Other factors such as sepsis and related inflammatory insults are examined. We explore recent studies implicating pro-inflammatory omega-6 fatty acids and the resulting encouraging trials with omega-3 fatty acids. Lastly, we discuss other damaging components of PN, including concerns about contaminants such as aluminum.

For each of the above mentioned theories of pathogenesis, multiple treatment methods have been proposed and attempted, but none alone has eliminated this disease. It is apparent that this multi-factorial issue will require a multi-faceted approach. We examine many of the attempted treatments and summarize their effectiveness, concluding with the most widely used and effective treatment regimes.

Introduction: Diagnosis, Incidence, and Risk Factors

Despite its instrumental role in neonatal care, PN is still responsible for considerable infant morbidity and even mortality. Since 1971, bile stasis and subsequent liver damage have become well-recognized and feared complications of PN in infants. [1,2] The following chapter will describe the theories of pathophysiology and corresponding treatments for this disease.

Diagnosis: Generally an infant must meet 3 criteria to be diagnosed with PNALD. These criteria are: biochemical evidence of liver dysfunction, dependence on PN and no other likely cause of cholestasis. [3,4] Hyperbilirubinemia, or a serum direct bilirubin greater than 2mg/dL (>34μmol/L) indicates early liver dysfunction and precedes any histologic evidence liver damage. [2,3,5] Direct bilirubin is the most commonly used biochemical indicator of PNALD, but it is often combined with measurements of liver transaminases, as direct bilirubin is not a perfect indicator. [6] Liver biopsy is the gold standard for diagnosing cholestasis, but is rarely performed due to its invasive nature.[4] PNALD is a diagnosis of exclusion and other causes of cholestasis must be ruled out, including: α1-antitrypsin deficiency, hypothyroidism, congenital infections, galactosemia, and metabolic disorders, along with extra-hepatic obstructions such as choledochal cysts and biliary atresia. [4,7]

Of note, although parenteral nutrition associated liver disease (PNALD) does not have exactly the same meaning as parenteral nutrition associated cholestasis (PNAC), or intestinal failure associated liver disease (IFALD) the terms are often used interchangeably. For this discussion PNALD will be used as it describes both the biliary stasis secondary to parenteral nutrition (PNAC) and the resulting long-term liver damage. [8]

Incidence: Considerable variation exists between reports on the incidence of PNALD, likely due to differing criteria for diagnosis. Generally however, 40-60% of all infants on long-term PN will develop some degree of cholestasis,[9,10] and when only infants with intestinal failure are considered, that statistic grows to 75%. [11] While at least one institute has published a decline in the incidence of PNALD, [12] corroborating reports comparing appropriate populations are not apparent.

Risk Factors: Prematurity is one of the most important risk factors for PNALD. Infants are more susceptible than adults to PNALD and premature infants especially are prone to poorer outcomes. [2,8,13,14] Low birth weight infants [15,16] or small for gestation age infants (SGA), are also at higher risk than those appropriate for gestational age (AGA). A few studies have found that cholestasis started earlier, was more severe and lasted longer in the SGA vs AGA. [17,18] One large population study reported that 39% of infants weighing less than 750gm developed PNALD. [19] These premature and smaller neonates may be at higher risk because of altered metabolic functioning of the liver, decreased glycogen stores and other forms of hepatobiliary underdevelopment.[18]

Additionally cited risk factors include surgical procedures or necrotizing enterocolitis (NEC) [8,13,14,19]; though these conditions coincide. One cohort study found that 70% of infants undergoing surgery for NEC later developed PNALD, [20] likely because this places the infant at highest risk of intestinal failure (and long-term PN dependence).[21] Odds ratios for the development of PNALD in patients with other commonly encountered pediatric diagnoses include gastroschisis (OR=20.3) and jejunal atresia (OR=24.0). [19]

Lastly, the duration of PN is important. No agreement on the length of time required to induce PNALD has been determined, but longer exposure increases the risks of cholestasis. [8,10,15,16,20,22] As an example, the Intermountain Healthcare NICUs (Utah, USA) report treating 9861 neonates and found that neonates receiving PN for 14-28 days had a 14% incidence of PNALD, with a worsening trend for longer duration. (43% incidence for 29-56 days, 72% for 57-100 days and 85% for >100 days). [19] Liver biopsies also support the importance of the duration of PN, where the first abnormalities are evident as early as two weeks and fulminant cirrhosis evident over the course of several months. [15] Most population studies report that 25% of infants on PN will develop some form of cholestasis within three weeks of exposure. [16,23] When infants on PN are followed for a longer period of time, almost all with more than sixty days of exposure will develop some degree of cholestasis. [3,24]

Histology

PNALD in infants is histologically heterogeneous, but is usually characterized by cholestasis and fibrosis. The former is a result of bile accumulating in both the canaliculi and hepatocytes, and is one of the most frequently noted findings. [15,16,22,25,26] Cholestasis is also one of the earliest histologic changes, and has been reported as soon as two weeks into PN exposure. [15] Bile canaliculi, when viewed by electron microscopy studies, show massive dilatation, lack of microvilli with bile plugging, and collagen in the space of Disse. [26] Generally, the centrilobular regions are the first site to display cholestasis, while fibrosis is usually first apparent in the periportal areas. Bile stasis triggers the later findings of fibrosis and ductal changes. [3] Fibrosis follows closely after cholestasis and its perivenular location allows for differentiation from other causes of hepatic fibrosis. [22] Eventually, the fibrosis may grow out from portal regions until there are fibrous bridges between each portal area. [3,26]

Beyond cholestasis and fibrosis, other signs of cellular and ductal injury are often present, such as extensive ballooning and feathering of the hepatocytes; occasionally progressing to apoptosis. [16,22] This lack of healthy cellular structure can lead to poor development of subsequent acini, such that small pseudoacinars form, without central veins. [3] Not surprisingly, with this degree of cell injury and death, inflammation is evident, with predominantly lymphatic peri-portal changes, and the occasional presence of giant cells. [26] This disordered inflammatory response may progress to the point where extramedullary hematopoiesis appears. [3,15,25,26] Eventually, a micronodular pattern of cirrhosis can be found in end-stage disease. [4]

The progression of ductal disease however, remains controversial. Traditionally, ductal proliferation has been present, [3,15,25] but more recent studies have found ductal retraction and ductopenia in the earlier stages of fibrosis. This suggests the possibility of a separate injury pathway coinciding with that of the fibrosis. [22]

Generally, children are more prone to developing fibrosis, while adults exposed to PN are more likely to develop steatosis of the liver. [15,16,22,25,27] For example, in a survey of PNALD in multiple age groups, Naini et al. (2012) reported that 60% of the those less than six months developed severe fibrosis, compared to only 19% in older children and adults. [22] Overall, the extent of hepatocellular damage appears to be inversely dependent on the age of the infant, with a greater progression of fibrosis to cirrhosis in the youngest age groups. [22,28]

Pathophysiology

Many pathophysiology theories explaining PNALD have been postulated, but it is accepted that the true cause of PNALD is likely multifactorial. Implicated factors can generally be grouped into those related to lack of physiologic enterohepatic circulation/enteric intake, those related to toxicity directly from the PN or its components, and those related to complications outside of the PN such as sepsis, need for gastrointestinal surgery, or other underlying co-morbidities. [5,13,29,30]

Immature Biliary System

Infants are born with an immature enterohepatic circulation of bile acids and, not surprisingly, preterm infants have even more problems handling bile acids. Normally bile acids are secreted from the hepatocytes into the bile canaliculi and then pass into the intestinal system through the biliary tree. The vast majority of bile acids are then reabsorbed in the ileum and travel back to the hepatocytes via the portal blood flow. [31] In the infant, however, many insufficiencies in this recirculation of bile exist, including failure to effectively resorb bile acids from the intestine and a reduced bile pool. [32,33]

Regardless of term, the newborn infant has poorly functioning active transport of bile acids in the ileum that results in bile salts being lost from the gastrointestinal tract. Often, this is compounded by bowel loss or malfunction, which further impairs reabsorption. [32] Even if reabsorption is successful, the bile acids are often trapped in the serum because neonatal hepatic extraction of bile acids from the serum is also impaired. [33] As a result of these inefficiencies, the overall bile pool is proportionally much smaller than it should be (when compared to a healthy adult). Bile acids provide positive feedback for bile flow in the liver, so the smaller bile pool leads to hepatic bile stasis. [34]

In premature infants, these above problems are made worse by a mismatch between formation and secretion of hepatic bile salts. Animal studies have shown synthesis of bile salts occurs much sooner than the efficient secretion of them, leading to a functional cholestasis in immature infants. [32] A more advanced secretion of bile acids has usually developed for those infants born at full term gestation, but it is incomplete even then. [32] The neonate, and especially the preterm neonate, is therefore at greater risk of cholestasis and PNALD because of these developmental issues.

Bile Acid Transporters BSEP, NTCP, OATP, MRP2 and Radixin

As described above, infants have deficiencies in almost all of the steps necessary for normal enterohepatic circulation of bile. This may be due to delayed development of bile acid transporter proteins and the nuclear transcription factors that control them. [35] Also possible is that the bile acid transporters may be poorly positioned in more immature livers. [36] Either insufficiency would hinder bile transport and predispose the newborn to cholestasis. The following sections will discuss bile transporters implicated in PNALD and other forms of neonatal cholestasis.

Note: traditionally human proteins are capitalized, while animal proteins have only the first letter capitalized.

BSEP: Bile salt export pump (also known as ABCB11) is one of the most important bile acid transporters, as it is positioned at the rate limiting step of biliary flow-excretion into the canaliculi. 37] It is found exclusively in the liver, on the canalicular membrane, and transports conjugated monovalent bile acids. [37] There is an almost 1000-fold difference in bile salt concentration gradients, so BSEP needs to be an active transporter to overcome this gradient and move bile salts out of the hepatocyte. [38] In fact, mutations in this protein lead to the devastating inherited disorder Progressive Familial Intrahepatic Cholestasis type 2, where cholestasis presents in infancy and progresses to cirrhosis and liver failure in the first ten years of life. [37,39,40] In contrast to rat pup studies, where this transporter may take up to 4 weeks to reach adult protein levels, studies of human fetal liver suggest that BSEP is expressed at 30-50% of adult levels but may not be properly localized until later in life. [35,36]

BSEP responds to many different cholestatic diseases through both transcriptional and post-transcriptional regulation. [37] Primary biliary cirrhosis is frequently used as a reference disease with elevated bile acids, and in this situation, BSEP has an indirect upregulatory effect, increasing both BSEP mRNA and protein levels. [37] In such situations, other BSEP transporters are also recruited from an intracellular pool, acting in response to increased bile acids, cAMP, and hypo-osmolarity. [37,41] These changes are likely an adaptation to improve clearance of bile acids from the hepatocyte. [42,43] However in other high bile acid scenarios, such as inflammation-induced cholestasis models, BSEP is decreased [44] and preliminary murine studies looking at BSEP in PNALD appear to correlate more with this model. [45] Further correlation in humans is still needed, as the murine Bsep does not seem to be quite as crucial as its human counterpart. [39]

MRP2: Multidrug resistance proteins are also ATP dependent transporters and there are four types located in the liver. MRP3 and MRP4 are found on the basolateral membrane, while MRP2 is solely on the apical, canalicular membrane. MRP1 is found in only very low levels in the liver. As a group, they export a variety of substrates into bile including glucuronidated (secondary) bile salts, estrogens, and glutathione conjugates of compounds. [46,47] Out of this family of transporters, MRP2 has the largest impact on biliary flow and transports bile acids out of the hepatocyte into the canaliculi. Similar to BSEP, fetal liver studies show 30-50% adult protein expression in the second trimester, as compared to rat studies where Mrp2 expression is delayed until 4 weeks after birth. [35,36] The fetal liver studies also found delayed positioning of the MRP2, but the pattern of MRP2 was more mature than fetal BSEP. [36]

Despite its importance in hepatobiliary function, many unanswered questions remain about the MRP2's role in different types of cholestasis. For example, mutations in this transporter create a surprisingly benign condition: Dubin-Johnson syndrome, characterized by conjugated hyperbilirubinemia with intact biliary excretion. [39] Although a few researchers have reported that MRP2 mRNA is increased in high bile states, [42,44] most others have found it to be decreased. [47,48] In particular, this has been found in a murine bile duct ligation model [47] and small population studies of primary biliary cirrhosis. [48] Similarly, PNALD models in mice have shown significant down-regulation of Mrp2 mRNA. [49,45] Interestingly, one was a 7 day model and Mrp2 downregulation was the only sign of hepatic dysregulation, implying that the alteration in bile transport proteins is an early sign, or precursor, to PNALD. [49]

For those proteins MRP2 and BSEP which are successfully expressed, oxidative stress can lead to additional damage in diseases such as PNALD. Preliminary evidence (extrapolated from other models of cholestasis) suggests that oxidative stress causes these bile export proteins to be internalized to a lysosomal compartment and possibly degraded. [46,50,51] The exact reasons for this relocation remain to be discerned; although the linker protein radixin may be involved.

Radixin: This linker protein likely connects the plasma membrane and transport proteins in the plasma membrane to the actin cytoskeleton of bile canalicular microvilli. [50] Co-localization studies of cholestasis have shown that both radixin and the bile acid protein MRP2 lose their normal co-localization, suggesting that the stabilization of radixin is necessary for normal canalicular positioning of export proteins. [50,52,53] Experiments with mice lacking radixin have provided further evidence for the relationship between radixin and export proteins. These animals developed the expected amount of Mrp2, however the protein was not in correct apical membrane position and the mice went on to develop conjugated hyperbilirubinemia. [54]

NTCP: Sodium-dependent taurocholic cotransporting polypeptide is another important transporter, which may play a role in PNALD. Located in the basolateral membrane of hepatocytes, NTCP carries bile acids into the cell from the portal blood stream (through the space of Disse). [39] NTCP has the highest affinity for conjugated bile acids, but is also known to transport unconjugated bile acids, sulfated bile acids, and steroid sulfates. As of yet, no disease process has been identified following the absence or mutation of this transporter. [55] However, some evidence suggests that functional impairment of this transporter may play a role in hypercholanemia. [55] Additionally, its expression has been shown to be decreased in high bile acid situations, perhaps as a defensive mechanism to limit the amount of toxic biliary products in the hepatocyte. [42,44] Similarly, pro-inflammatory cytokines and endotoxins (such as are found in PNALD) indirectly down-regulate both mRNA and protein levels of NTCP. [37,43,56] This inflammation triggered down-regulation could play a role in PNALD, but evidence for this is currently lacking. [39]

OATP: Organic anion transporting polypeptides (OATP), like NTCP, are also found on the basolateral membrane, but differ in that they are responsible for the entry of unconjugated bile acids into the hepatocyte. [39,57] A collection of members of the OATP family are found in the liver with subtly different functions. Generally OATPs transport large anionic amphipathic molecules, but a few types can transport enzymes such as cholecystokinin 8 and even cations. [39,57] Based on rat studies, OATP development is suspected to occur even later than BSEP and NTCP. [57]

Similar to NTCP, no disease has yet been identified secondary to mutations in this transporter. However, elevated bile acids have varying effects on the different members of the OATP family. For example, humans with primary sclerosing cholangitis have decreased expression of some subtypes of OATP, with increased expression of others. [39] OATP2 in particular, has been studied extensively and is decreased in later stages of primary biliary cirrhosis and inflammation-induced cholestasis. [42,43,44,48] Similar to NTCP, researchers have theorized that OATP likely plays a role in PNALD and other acquired cholestasis based on its role in inflammation-induced cholestasis models. [44]

Enteral Stasis

As early as 1975, the lack of enteral stimulation was correlated with the development of cholestasis, and prolonged fasting was later proposed to contribute to disruptions in bile flow. [3,34] Bile acid secretion is proportional to oral intake, and the lack of enteral stimulation also decreases many important gastrointestinal and hepatic hormones, such as cholecystokinin, gastrin, motilin, secretin, pancreatic polypeptide, glucagon, and vasoactive intestinal peptide. [29,33] Cholecystokinin deficits in particular, may lead to reduced gallbladder contractility and impediment of the enterohepatic circulation. [30,33] In addition, the liver must adapt to changes in portal flow, because the nutrients are now delivered through the arterial system instead of through the portal vein. This inversion of nutrient blood flow places unexpected demands on the acini, as zones unaccustomed to the exposure of nutrient-rich blood become the first to filter it, essentially reversing the zones of filtration. [30]

Enteral feeding is known to have other benefits in PN-dependent patients, such as enhancing gut motility and adaptation. [58] In murine models, even if PN is given enterally, it restores blood flow to the small intestine and portal vein. It may also improve the hepatic immune response, thereby combating the reduction in both intestinal blood flow and hepatic immune function seen in animal models of PN. This same research group has also demonstrated that PN given enterally does not depress the hepatic immune response, supporting the idea that it is the absence of gut stimulation that is damaging. [59] Given the damaging effects of fasting and the benefits to enteral stimulation, most critical care units promote enteral feeding as early as safely possible. [58]

Sepsis

Sepsis has long been correlated with PNALD as those infants with multiple septic events have a higher incidence of cholestasis. [10,60] The liver plays a key role in the inflammatory response to invading pathogens, even when the primary site of infection is extrahepatic. [61] Kupffer cells (liver macrophages), hepatocytes, and biliary epithelium all release cytokines (TNF-a, IL-1 etc.), nitric oxide, and other mediators to boost the pro-inflammatory cascade. [61,62] Unfortunately, with activation of the inflammatory response, reactive oxygen radicals are often produced and surrounding hepatocytes may be damaged. In turn, accumulation of nitric oxide may lead to vascular collapse, further damaging the liver and leading to necrosis. [62]

In addition, decreased bowel function may impair immune function because the gastrointestinal lymphoid tissue is negatively affected. [30] This bowel and immune stasis places the patient at risk of bacterial overgrowth [60] and translocation. [10,29] As opposed to common extrahepatic infections such as line sepsis, bowel stasis induces a gram negative, anaerobic bacterial sepsis. The link between anaerobic bacteria and cholestasis has been suggested in studies such as Lambert et al. [60] who described a rise in liver enzymes in patients on PN without metronidazole prophylaxis, compared to those who received the antibiotic. Given that metronidazole suppresses intestinal anaerobic bacteria, the authors postulated that this type of bacteria contributes to hepatic injury.[60] Others have likewise reported that infants with sepsis and cholestasis are more likely to have gram negative cultures. [18] Gram negative bacteria (such as E.coli) produces damaging lipopolysaccharides which can reduce the expression of export pumps BSEP and MRP2. [61] Direct hepatic damage is also caused by endotoxins and toxic bile salts released from intestinal bacteria. [61] Specific work examining lipopolysaccharides has shown that both a lack of enteral feeding and bacterial overgrowth is needed for these toxic substances to reach the liver. [63] Once these substances reach the liver in sufficient amounts they activate the Toll-like receptors in Kupffer cells setting off the localized inflammatory cascade as described above. [63]

Regardless of the source of bacteria, the liver is at risk during septic episodes due to its natural immune functions and the dysregulation of these functions caused by PN.

Elemental Components/Contaminants of PN: Manganese, Copper, Aluminum

Manganese, copper, and other trace elements have all been investigated and varying results have led to debate over the protocol for adding them to infant PN. [10] Currently, zinc supplementation is the only trace element that must be given with the initiation of PN in the infant, and all other trace elements can be added 2-4 weeks later. Due to the contaminants in PN, adding trace elements can be difficult, as the infant may already be exposed to manganese and copper contaminants outside of the regulated addition. [64]

Manganese: Although manganese is an essential element, few cases of clinical deficiency have been reported. More commonly, manganese is toxic, causing Parkinson-like neurologic symptoms. As it is excreted via the biliary system, any infant with cholestasis is at risk for accumulation of this element; especially since manganese has a 100% bioavailability when delivered intravenously. [64] It also appears that the youngest patients are least able to excrete this element and accumulate the highest levels, likely secondary to their immature hepatobiliary system. [65,66]

However, the evidence for manganese contributing to cholestasis is still developing. A study of PN-dependent children found manganese levels to be correlated with serum bilirubin levels, AST and cholestasis. When manganese was reduced in these children, the bilirubin fell accordingly, but the AST appeared slower to respond. [65] The cause and effect is still uncertain, but the manganese may accumulate secondary to liver disease and then worsen the hepatic damage. Controversy also exists regarding the presence of manganese contamination, with some studies finding contamination [67,66] and others stating there is virtually none. [65] In response, the European Society for Clinical Nutrition and Metabolism and other expert organizations advise a reduced amount of manganese supplementation, and many institutions now remove manganese in infants with PNALD. [68,69]

Copper: Similar to manganese, copper is excreted primarily through the biliary system, placing cholestatic infants at risk of copper toxicity. [64] However, there is very little evidence that copper toxicity actually causes the cholestasis and the available studies have been performed in adults. Blaszyk et al. (2005) found that one third of adult patients on long term PN accumulated serum copper levels above the threshold for diagnosing Wilson's disease (a disease of copper overload secondary to a genetic defect in biliary clearance). The hepatic copper levels also correlated with the serum total and direct bilirubin. Interestingly, in this study the copper overload appeared to have no relationship to the duration of TPN, instead it correlated with the sickest individuals. This led the authors to conclude that copper accumulation is a result of the cholestasis (inability of the liver to clear copper) as opposed to the cause of cholestasis. [70] As a precaution, it is recommended that copper levels be monitored closely, [68] and those patients with cholestasis may need to have copper reduced in their trace elements to avoid toxicity. [8,68]

Aluminum: While aluminum has no role in human physiology and thus cases of aluminum deficiency do not exist, many cases of aluminum toxicity have been described. This is especially true in PN-dependent patients as much higher amounts are absorbed systemically when aluminum is given parenterally as opposed to the <1% absorbed in oral ingestion. [71] This is problematic, as high doses of aluminum cause anemia, neurologic disorders, and impaired bone metabolism [72].

In 2004, United States Food and Drug Administration (FDA) recommended that aluminum intake be < 5μg/kg/day [73], while the American Society for Parenteral and Enteral Nutrition (ASPEN) stated that 15-30μg/kg/day is unsafe, and 60μg/kg/day toxic. [74] Large volume PN solutions (dextrose and amino acids) must contain less than 25μg/L of aluminum, but a lack of regulation for small volume PN products makes it difficult to regulate total aluminum intake. [73] Actual analysis of the aluminum in infant PN has revealed levels three to five times greater than the FDA limit. [71] Of concern, the highest levels of aluminum have been found in the smallest infants on PN. [71]

A wide collection of PN components are contaminated with aluminum, including amino acids, dextrose solutions, lipid emulsions, trace elements, multivitamins, heparin, and insulin, but the majority is found in calcium gluconate, potassium phosphate and sodium phosphate. These latter compounds become contaminated by forming complex ions with the aluminum leeched out of their glass containers. [71,75] Infants accumulate aluminum because much more calcium gluconate in particular, is required for growth as compared to adults. [75,76] The third trimester is the time of calcium accretion, and therefore preterm infants require even greater amounts of supplemental calcium to avoid osteopenia of prematurity. [77] Premature infants also have immature renal function and since aluminum is excreted via the renal pathway, the toxicity is compounded. [71,76]

Since the early 1980s, researchers have identified high aluminum levels in infants with PNALD, but the link between the element and disease is not yet fully understood. [78-81] Animal models have provided some clues, for instance, rats exposed to high doses of aluminum developed elevated bile acid levels, with evidence that sinusoidal uptake and canalicular excretion was impaired. [46,82] (Of note, these changes occur despite enteral feeding). [82] Histological changes including portal inflammation, and aluminum-laden giant cells have also been found following aluminum exposure, [83,84] but plasma membrane changes were not initially detected until very large doses (1500μg/kg/day) were used. [78] These changes included blunted bile canalicular microvilli, a decreased number of microvilli, and dilatation of the canaliculi. [78]

Alemmari et al. (2012) conducted a study with newborn pigs to further investigate whether histological changes could be seen with PN aluminum contamination closer to the level seen in clinical settings. This resulted in more significant changes to the bile canalicular microvilli in the regular PN group vs an experimentally low aluminum PN group. [79] Further evidence for aluminum affecting the plasma membrane comes from studies where rats exposed to high amounts of aluminum developed a 40% decreased expression of Mrp2, and similar results have been replicated in our laboratory using piglets. [46, Alemmari et al. (2011 unpublished)] The mechanism of injury may be through oxidative stress, because this element causes oxidative stress through multiple pathways. For example, aluminum forms aluminum superoxide, it participates in other oxidative reactions with iron, and it causes mitochondria to leak electrons (increasing radical oxygen species). [85] In addition, aluminum increases lipid peroxidation. [85].

Given this evidence, aluminum does appear to impede biliary flow and may do so through changes at the canalicular plasma membrane. Based on the known toxicity of aluminum, the UK Medicines and Healthcare Products Regulatory Agency has already taken steps to reduce contamination in PN, by restricting the use of glass vials for small volume PN products. [86] Health Canada has recently published similar concerns about the hepatotoxic/neurotoxic effect of aluminum in glass vials, and a warning is now printed on the package inserts for calcium gluconate in Canada. [87,88]

Macronutrient Components of PN: Amino Acids, Glucose and Lipids

Amino acids: In the early 1980s there was concern around overfeeding secondary to PN protein content. It was postulated that excess amino acids may be a direct hepatic toxin and impair bile flow. [89] One study compared high (3.6gm/kg/day) vs low protein (2.3gm/kg/day) and found that although there was a similar number of cholestatic cases in each group, those with the higher protein developed cholestasis earlier (27 versus 47 days), and achieved a greater peak direct bilirubin. [89]

In the subsequent decades, due to infant-specific fomulations, amino acid provision has become less of an issue.[68,90] More recent studies have found no evidence that the current amount of protein or amino acid (approximately 2.5gm/kg/day) [91] places an infant at risk of cholestasis. [90,91]

Glucose: Early research into PNALD also suggested that glucose overload may be hepatotoxic, and it was recommended by some authors that one third of the glucose calories should be replaced by lipids. [92] This recommendation was based on studies from the 1980s in adults which demonstrated half the level of liver enzymes in patients with 15% dextrose vs 50%. [92] Concurrent research identified a similar correlation between higher dextrose levels and cholestasis but more recent work has disputed the theory that glucose is responsible for PNALD. (Although over-feeding is still cautioned against). [68,93] Attention has instead turned to the influence of lipids.

Lipids: After a flurry of recent research, lipids have emerged as one of the most plausible contributors in the pathophysiology of PNALD. There are two theories explaining the damaging effects of lipids: the phytosterol content and the pro-inflammatory nature of omega-6 vs omega-3 fatty acids.

Phytosterols: Phytosterols are derived from plant-based lipid sources (traditionally soy) and are almost identical to cholesterol, with matching nuclei but different alkylated side chains. [94] Traditionally available intravenous lipids are usually soy-based and contain the phytosterols sitosterol, campesterol, and stigmasterol at a total concentration of approximately

1000μmol/L (40 mg/dL). [95] In comparison, fish oils (i.e., Omegaven™) do not contain any phytosterols [96] and olive-oil based lipids have fewer than soy-based emulsions. [97]

Many studies have found an increase in serum plant sterol levels in patients receiving PN [97] and animal models have exhibited both an increase in bile acids with infusion of phytosterols, and subsequent reversal of bilirubin with reduction of phytosterols. [98] For example, piglets injected with sterols at a similar level as seen clinically in PN developed significantly higher level of serum bile acids and reduced bile flow. [94]

Phytosterols are only excreted via the biliary system, but hepatic metabolism of these compounds is very slow. In fact, the degrading enzyme 7α-hydroxylase has a 30 fold greater affinity for cholesterol vs the phytosterol sitosterol. [99] During this prolonged exposure, phytosterols are thought to replace the cholesterol in the cell membranes and interfere with bile acid transport proteins. [99,100] For instance, phytosterols hinder the nuclear receptor farnesoid X, a key regulator of bile acid production. [97,98]

However high phytosterol levels may be a consequence rather than the causation of PNALD. Case reports have shown at least some phytosterols falling with reduction of glucose rather than lipids, perhaps implying that phytosterols are an indicator of liver dysfunction rather than lipid toxicity. [95] A recent study examining the use of five different types of lipid emulsions in neonates also found no association between phytosterol intake and liver function at six weeks of exposure. Of particular interest is the observation that in the group with the highest phytosterol intake, there were no cases of cholestasis. [101] These findings support the current theory that omega-6 fatty acids contribute more than phytosterols to the pathophysiology of PNALD. [8]

Omega-6 vs omega-3 fatty acids: Omega-6 fatty acids (as found in soy-based emulsions) are pro-inflammatory, and likely hepatotoxic, making them one of the key factors in PNALD development. [102-104] This group of polyunsaturated fats includes linoleic acid and arachidonic acid, compared to the omega-3 fatty acids group which includes docosahexaenoic acid, alpha-linolenic acid, and eicospentanoic acid. [105] The pro-inflammatory effects of omega-6 fatty acids are secondary to their production of platelet aggregating thromboxanes and formation of immunosuppressing prostaglandin E1 (through arachidonic acid). In addition, soy-based preparations have very little α-tocopherol (absorbable vitamin E) to combat these inflammatory effects. [106] Meanwhile, omega-3 fatty acids appear to be hepatoprotective, with anticoagulating thromboxanes and the formation of prostaglandin E3 to assist immune function. [96,103,104] Omega-3 fatty acids may also help to regulate tumour necrosis factor-α, known to be damaging in sepsis. [96] Having gained further understanding into these mechanisms, many groups have proposed a switch from the traditional omega-6 fatty acids lipids to omega-3 lipid emulsions and the results of these trials will be covered in the subsequent section on treatments of PNALD.

A switch to omega-3 fatty acids does raise concerns, as these fatty acids represent a markedly different composition than human milk lipids, and omega-6 fatty acids are needed to act as building blocks for the essential fatty acid alpha-linoleic. [101,103] Caution must therefore be exercised in selecting lipid solutions, to avoid essential fatty acid deficiency and subsequent impairment in brain development. Both omega-6 linoleic acid and omega-3 alpha-linoleic acid are customarily designated as essential fatty acids. [105] Newer work has since questioned this strict designation and some authors have suggested that in low-birth weight infants, there may be additional essential fatty acids. Low-birth weight infants are unable to convert linoleic and alpha-linoleic acid to arachidonic, eicospentanoic, and docosahexaenoic acid and therefore an omega-3 lipid solution may be better, as it provides these downstream fatty acids (although only small amounts of arachidonic acid). [104,105]

In response to concerns of essential fatty acid deficiency, mixtures of omega-3 and omega-6 fatty acids have been developed, i.e.: SMOFlipid™ (soybean/MCT/olive/fish emulsion)(Fresenius Kabi). [106] As well as providing both traditional and conditionally essential fatty acids, this mixture also has a higher level of α-tocopherol to combat lipid peroxidation (200mg/L in SMOFlipid™, vs 38 in Intralipid™). [106,107]

Critics of the lipid contribution to PNALD point to a collection of studies that have failed to find a correlation between lipids and cholestasis in infants. [20,89] Similarly, PNALD was reported before the widespread use of lipids into standard PN and this discrepancy has not yet been explained. [80] Given the positive results of lipid trials (see Treatment section), lipids clearly play a role in pathogenesis, but it is crucial to remember that this is a multi-factorial disease and benefits from a variety of treatment approaches.

Treatments

Since a variety of factors contribute to the pathophysiology of this disease, the best results in treatment have also been multi-factorial. [21] An additional aspect of successful treatment appears to be the use of a multidisciplinary team within a regional treatment site. [7,21,108] The following section will further explore each treatment individually, but important to remember is that these therapies are used in combination for best results.

Enteral feeding: Cholestasis only completely resolves once the infant is on enteral feeds and no longer receiving PN. [109] Switching to enteral feeding is therefore the most effective treatment, as it often brings about clinical and biochemical improvement within 2 weeks. [26] Unfortunately, attempts to wean infants off of PN are fraught with problems due to their complicated medical condition. Often these infants cannot tolerate substantial enteral nutrition and instead can only be given small amounts in hopes of stimulating the bowel. This has proven beneficial to gut function, [58,59] and is commonly practiced in critical care units, but does not reliably prevent PNALD. [109]

Cycling: This is routinely performed by some institutions after an infant has been on PN for at least 2 weeks. [68] The protocol involves adjusting the rate of infusion so that PN is given in a shorter time period, thereby allowing the liver to rest. [110] In infants this must be carried out cautiously to avoid micro and macro nutrient deficiencies because they have limited reserve. [9] In particular, neonates are vulnerable to extremes of glucose as they have not yet developed reliable methods of glucose homeostasis. [111] Moreover, cycling may increase line sepsis because of the frequent line access required. If performed carefully, prophylactic cycling does appear to postpone PNALD, but multiple studies have shown that by itself it does not prevent eventual cholestasis. [112,113]

Ursodeoxycholic acid (UDCA): One of the most logical approaches to a faulty enterohepatic circulation is to directly alter bile secretion. Accordingly, agents such as UDCA have been used, but with varying success. UDCA is taken up by the liver and conjugated into a functional bile acid, which is then secreted back into the bile and works to aid in fat digestion. It increases the bile acid-dependent bile flow and promotes enterohepatic circulation, and is also believed to decrease the hydrophobic content of bile, making it less damaging to biliary epithelium [114]. Early studies showed resolution of deranged liver enzymes and bilirubin within 4-8weeks of UDCA, with rebound of enzymes when the UDCA was discontinued. However, the dosage used in this study was higher than recommended, [115] and subsequent clinical results have been mixed, with some showing no benefit and others only modest improvement. [116-118] These studies are often hard to interpret due to confounders such as the concurrent use of enteral feeding and small number of infants. [8] Others have raised concerns about the safety of administering doses large enough to stimulate a noticeable increase in bile secretion. [33] In contrast, chenodeoxycholic acid is a similar compound which acts to restore normal enterohepatic circulation through its effects on bile acid regulators. It appears to effect a wider range of receptors than UDCA and although investigations into this compound are only preliminary, results are encouraging. [119]

Cholecystokinin octopeptide: This enzyme causes gallbladder contraction and stimulation of bile flow and thus, was expected to produce positive effects in PNALD. Unfortunately, this has been refuted in a large trial demonstrating no prevention of cholestasis or gallstones in those infants on PN. [118,120] Although some reports of cholecystokinin preventing PNALD in the adult population exist, this has not translated into the neonatal population because of differences in hepatic maturity and enterohepatic circulation. [120]

Taurine: This amino acid has been considered as a potential treatment because children on long term PN are often taurine deficient, and infants are known to be less efficient at converting methionine and cysteine into taurine. [121,122] A paucity of taurine means that the preferable taurine-conjugated bile acids cannot be formed and instead, the more toxic and hydrophobic glycine-conjugated bile acids are created. [123] However, not all animal studies have borne out this theory, as rats with higher levels of taurine supplementation have shown the greatest impairment in drug clearance (85% reduction as compared to the non-PN group). [122] It does appears to have at least modest benefits in infants, although not for all groups. One large study demonstrated a trend in decreased incidence of cholestasis within very premature infants, and a significantly reduced incidence in those with NEC. Although results are not conclusive, many hospitals now use amino-acid mixtures containing taurine; with the added benefit that it is important for retinal development. [121]

Antibiotics: Empiric antibiotics are often initiated in situations of sepsis-associated cholestasis, [62] and metronidazole in particular has been proposed as a 'bowel decontaminant' to decrease bacterial overgrowth and translocation, as well as to prevent production of toxic, cholestatic bile salts. [61,110]

However, the results are not conclusive and the American Pediatric Surgical Association's position is that evidence is not sufficient to support routine prophylactic use of antibiotics to prevent PNALD. [8]

Interestingly, probiotics were used in a PN rabbit model in an attempt to control bacterial overgrowth of the intestine and reduce endotoxemia. This resulted in significantly lower levels of total bilirubin and bile acid with improved bowel and liver histology. The bacterial translocation rate was also slowed and endotoxins decreased. Further research in this area may clarify the relationship between sepsis and PNALD. [124]

Lipid modification: Until very recently, only one lipid emulsion (Intralipid™, Baxter/Fresenius Kabi, Deerfield, IL, USA) was used by most North American institutions due to difficulty in obtaining approval for other formulations. [104] However, other emulsions are slowly coming into practice, often through compassionate use programs or investigational new drug applications. [104,125] The following sections will discuss approaches to modify lipid amounts and emulsion types.

Lipid reduction: Although lipid reduction is an appealing method of decreasing an infant's exposure to pro-inflammatory omega-6 fatty acids, it must be carried out cautiously as lipids are a critical source of energy in this population. While the average person is at risk of essential fatty acid deficiency if essential fatty acids are less than 1-2% of the total caloric intake, premature infants require twice this amount for healthy growth and neurologic development. [126] Infants can display the biochemical changes of deficiency within a few days of deprivation. [105,126] One reason for this susceptibility is that even if extra glucose (and therefore insulin) is given to stimulate triglycerides, these triglycerides cannot be released without essential fatty acids. [127]

Preliminary studies in infants indicate that Intralipid 20%, which is often given in doses of up to 3 gm/kg/day [104] could be safely reduced to 1-2gm/kg/day with careful monitoring. The results of at least one such study in infants with cholestasis have shown a reversal of serum bilirubin levels without the development of irreversible essential fatty acid deficiency. In this group, increased dextrose was given to ensure adequate energy supply and growth. Of note, a small proportion of infants did develop mild essential fatty acid deficiency (indicated by a triene:tetraene ratio >0.5 but <0.2) and required a subsequent increase in lipids. [103] For the most part, studies have looked at reducing lipids once the infant has developed cholestasis. But one group has looked to prevent the development of PNALD by decreasing the soy-based lipids from 2-3gm/kg/day to 1 gm/kg/day. This resulted in a significantly reduced level of direct bilirubin and 1.77 less risk of PNALD in those infants with a reduced level of lipids. [128] Overall, reduction of lipids is used by some groups, but cautiously and usually after the development of PNALD.

Lipids-Fish-oil monotherapy: Omegaven™ (Fresenius Kabi, Bad Homburg, Germany) is a 10% fish-oil emulsion providing only polyunsaturated omega-3 fatty acids and although it is currently difficult to access in North America, results of its use in PNALD are favourable. In studies with fish oil monotherapy in infants with established PNALD, the serum direct bilirubin normalized and clinical status has improved for the majority of patients.[96,102,129,130] For example, in a study of 67 infants with PNALD who were switched to fish-oil monotherapy, it was observed that 82.5% had reversal of their serum bilirubin and survived to be discharged from hospital. [131] In addition, overall morbidity and mortality for infants with PNALD is substantially reduced on this formulation. [105,132]

Critics of this therapy have expressed concerns that an omega-3 emulsion alone would place an infant at risk of essential fatty acid deficiency. It has been pointed out that although triene/tetraene ratios may be normal, concentrations of individual fatty acids may still be dangerously low as fatty acid profiles are rarely reported. [125] Researchers working with Omegaven™ in large retrospective studies have argued that despite these concerns, careful monitoring for essential fatty deficiency has shown that the mixture of fatty acids in Omegaven™ is sufficient. [104,105] For example, more than 130 children in Boston have been treated with Omegaven™ and none of these patients developed clinical (growth retardation or dermatitis) or biochemical evidence (elevated triene–tetraene ratio) of essential fatty acid deficiency. [105,126] A separate group of 67 infants on fish oil emulsions also failed to show any evidence of essential fatty acid deficiency. [131] Regardless of these clinical findings, the manufacturer of Omegaven™ does not recommend the use of fish-oil based emulsions as a monotherapy, reiterating concerns about the low levels of the essential linoleic acid (0.1-0.7%). [105]

The debate about essential fatty acid deficiency secondary to Omegaven™ is ongoing even as its use becomes more widespread. Despite its successes, fish-oil is not a universal cure for all patients, as most studies include a small proportion of patients who do not improve. [96,102,125,129,130] In particular, it does not appear to be as successful with more advanced stages of disease and premature infants may be less responsive. [96,131,108] It is also not approved for use in North America.

Lipids-Omega-3 and 6 mixture: The newest lipid emulsion attempts to address concerns about essential fatty acid deficiency and pro-inflammatory omega-6 fatty acids. SMOFlipid™ (soybean/MCT/olive/fish emulsion) (Fresenius Kabi) [106] provides a mixture of lipids from multiple sources, and although it is a recent product, it is quickly becoming favoured. Initial studies in adults showed that SMOFlipid™ maintained normal liver enzymes and lower total bilirubin levels. [106,133] Likewise, a separate trial in children also found decreases in total bilirubin, as well as increased levels of serum α-tocopherol in the SMOFlipid™ as opposed to traditional lipid group. [107] A similar report focused on small groups of children with established PNALD on Intralipid™, half of whom were then switched to SMOFlipid™, with no reduction in the amount of lipid provided. At six months of treatment, cholestasis had resolved in five of eight in the SMOFlipid™ group, compared to only two of nine in the Intralipid™ group. In fact, the mean total bilirubin in the Intralipid™ group continued to increase throughout the study period by 79μmol/L compared to a decrease of 99μmol/L in the SMOFlipid™ group. Of note, multiple other treatment methods (cycling, UDCA etc.) were also used, as is routine in that centre. [7] In summary, the results of these trials are promising, but the American Society for Parenteral and Enteral Nutrition has stated that further research needs to be done to clearly define when alternative lipid emulsions (such as SMOFlipid™) are of most benefit. [134]

Other potential treatments: A multitude of other potential treatments are currently being investigated with varying results. For example, human growth factor has been used in PN-dependent rats with short bowel in an attempt to enhance the function of the remaining bowel, and although this did not affect the grade of hepatic inflammation or the bilirubin level, it did preserve the ductal system and reduce the apoptotic index. [135]

Immunosuppressants and immunomodulators are also being examined based on the theory that cytokines play an important role in the development of PNALD. For instance, PN-dependent mice given Infliximab (a TNF-α antibody) demonstrated improved liver histology and expression of bile acid transporter genes. Total and direct bilirubin levels also improved in the Infliximab mice compared to the PN+no Infliximab group. [45] Likewise IFN-α supplementation (an immunomodulator with anti-fibrotic effects) has shown that it may be beneficial in treating cholestasis. [136]

Long Term Consequences

For the majority of infants, PNALD is temporary and resolves after the discontinuation of PN. [5] For those children fortunate enough to recuperate from the hepatic damage, the recovery period (indicated by normal bilirubin levels) is two to four months. [9,109] Conversely, for the subset of infants who cannot be weaned off of PN, the initial cholestasis may lead to portal hypertension, cirrhosis, and end-stage liver disease requiring a transplant of the liver and/or bowel.

Direct bilirubin levels are often used as an indicator of prognosis, with higher levels correlated with worse outcomes. [9] Should the disease progress to a direct bilirubin >11mg/dL there is a 26% mortality rate. [19] Prolonged hyperbilirubinemia also has a poor prognosis. For instance, a large referral center for intestinal failure-associated liver disease found that if normalization of bilirubin levels could be achieved within one year of referral, the mortality and transplantation rates were 5.2%. But if the hyperbilirubinemia could not be reversed in this time period, the mortality and transplantation rates were 58%. [21]

For those infants who are successfully weaned off of PN, biochemical abnormalities usually resolve, but there may be long-standing liver damage,[26] and in some cases it may continue to progress. For example, although cholestasis had resolved, fibrosis and steatosis have been found on liver biopsies 8 years after stopping PN. In fact, the degree of fibrosis was similar to that of infants still reliant on PN. [28] This implies that some of these patients may develop a degree of compensated cirrhosis, and they must then be monitored for later potential malignancies. [6]

Conclusion

Many other aspects of neonatal care have improved since the first appearance of PNALD over forty years ago, but the concerns about prolonged PN and PNALD remain. This is a disease which affects the smallest and sickest infants, and the sequelae of PNALD can be devastating. Fortunately, better understanding of the pathophysiology has led to more effective treatments. PNALD is clearly a multi-factorial disease, where an immature hepatic system with a poorly functioning bowel then incurs injury from a collection of sources: sepsis, contaminants, and pro-inflammatory lipids. The most successful treatment regimens address this complex pathophysiology, often in specialized referral centers with multidisciplinary teams. Currently cycling of PN, prompt treatment of infections, maximizing enteral stimulation, UDCA, limited lipids, and using omega-3 (or mixed emulsions) appear to give these infants the most favourable outcomes. Further research will continue to broaden our understanding of this complex condition.

References

[1] Peden, V; Witzleben, C; Skelton, M; et al. Total parenteral nutrition. *J Pediatr*, 1971, 78, 180.

[2] Touloukian, RJ; Seashore, JH. Hepatic secretory obstruction with total parenteral nutrition in the infant. *J Pediatr Surg*, 1975, 10, 353-360.

[3] Benjamin, DR. Hepatobiliary dysfunction in infants and children associated with long-term total parenteral nutrition: a clinicopathologic study. *Am J Clin Pathol*, 1981, 76, 276-83.

[4] Mullick, FG; Moran, CA; Ishak, KG. Total parenteral nutrition: a histopathologic analysis of the liver changes in 20 children. *Mod Pathol*, 1994, 7, 190-4.

[5] Koseesirikul, P; Chotinaruemol, S; Ukarapol, N. Incidence and risk factors of parenteral nutrition-associated liver disease in newborn infants. *Pediatrics International*, 2012, 54(3), 434-6.

[6] Fitzgibbons, SC; Jones, BA; Hull, MA; Zurakowski, D; Duro, D; Duggan, C; et al. Relationship between biopsy-proven parenteral nutrition-associated liver fibrosis and biochemical cholestasis in children with short bowel syndrome. *Journal of Pediatric Surgery*, 2010, 45(1), 95-9.

[7] Muhammed, R; Bremner, R; Protheroe, S; Johnson, T; Holden, C; Murphy, MS. Resolution of parenteral nutrition-associated jaundice on changing from a soybean oil emulsion to a complex mixed-lipid emulsion. *Journal of Pediatric Gastroenterology & Nutrition*, 2012, 54(6), 797-802.

[8] Rangel, SJ; Calkins, CM; Cowles, RA; Barnhart, DC; Huang, EY; Abdullah, F; Arca, MJ; Teitelbaum, DH. For the 2011 American Pediatric Surgical Association Outcomes and Clinical Trials Committee. Parenteral nutrition–associated cholestasis: an American Pediatric Surgical Association Outcomes and Clinical Trials Committee systematic review. *Journal of Pediatric Surgery*, 2012, 47(1), 225-240.

[9] Willis, TC; Carter, BA; Rogers, SP; Hawthorne, KM; Hicks, PD; Abrams, SA. High rates of mortality and morbidity occur in infants with parenteral nutrition-associated cholestasis. *JPEN*, 2010, 34, 32-7.

[10] Suita, S; Masumoto, K; Yamanouchi, T; Nagano, M; Nakamura, M. Complications in neonates with short bowel syndrome and long-term parenteral nutrition. *J Parenter Enteral Nutr*, 1999, 23, S106-9.

[11] Squires, RH; Duggan, C; Teitelbaum, DH; et al. Pediatric Intestinal Failure Consortium. Natural history of pediatric intestinal failure: initial report from the Pediatric Intestinal Failure Consortium. *J Pediatr*, 2012, 161, 723–728.

[12] Kubota, A; Yonekura, T; Hoki, M; Oyanagi, H; Kawahara, H; Yagi, M; et al. Total parenteral nutrition-associated intrahepatic cholestasis in infants, 25 years' experience. *Journal of Pediatric Surgery*, 2000, 35(7), 1049-51.

[13] Beath, SV; Davies, P; Papadopoulou, A; et al. Parenteral nutrition-related cholestasis in postsurgical neonates: Multivariate analysis of risk factors. *J. Pediatr. Surg.,* 1996, 31, 604–6.

[14] Javid, PJ; Malone, FR; Dick, AA; Hsu, E; Sunseri, M; Healey, P; Horslen, SP. A contemporary analysis of parenteral nutrition-associated liver disease in surgical infants. *Journal of Pediatric Surgery*, 2011, 46(10), 1913-7.

[15] Zambrano, E; El-Hennawy, M; Ehrenkranz, RA; Zelterman, D; Reyes-Mugica, M. Total parenteral nutrition induced liver pathology: an autopsy series of 24 newborn cases. *Pediatric & Developmental Pathology*, 2004, 7(5), 425-32.

[16] Beale, EF; Nelson, RM; Bucciarelli, RL; Donnelly, WH; Eitzman, DV. Intrahepatic cholestasis associated with parenteral nutrition in premature infants. *Pediatrics*, 1979, 64(3), 342-7.

[17] Lee, SM; Namgung, R; Park, MS; Eun, HS; Kim, NH; Park, KI; Lee, C. Parenteral nutrition associated cholestasis is earlier, more prolonged and severe in small for gestational age compared with appropriate for gestational age very low birth weight infants. *Yonsei Medical Journal*, 2013, 54(4), 839-44.

[18] Robinson, DT; Ehrenkranz, RA. Parenteral nutrition–associated cholestasis in small for gestational age infants. *J Pediatr*, 2008, 152(1), 59-62.

[19] Christensen, RD; Henry, E; Wiedmeier, SE; et al. Identifying patients, on the first day of life, at high-risk of developing parenteral nutrition–associated liver disease. *J Perinatol*, 2007, 27(5), 284-90.

[20] Duro, D; Mitchell, PD; Kalish, LA; Martin, C; McCarthy, M; Jaksic, T; et al. Risk factors for parenteral nutrition-associated liver disease following surgical therapy for necrotizing enterocolitis: A Glaser Pediatric Research Network Study [corrected].[Erratum appears in J Pediatr Gastroenterol Nutr. 2011 Nov, 53(5): 583] *Journal of Pediatric Gastroenterology & Nutrition*, 2011, 52(5), 595-600.

[21] Cowles, RA; Ventura, KA; Martinez, M; et al. Reversal of intestinal failure–associated liver disease in infants and children on parenteral nutrition: experience with 93 patients at a referral center for intestinal rehabilitation. *J Pediatr Surg*, 2010, 45(1), 84-7.

[22] Naini, BV; Lassman, CR. Total parenteral nutrition therapy and liver injury: a histopathologic study with clinical correlation. *Human Pathology*, 2012, 43(6), 826-833

[23] Arnold, CJ. Thesis: Parenteral nutrition associated cholestasis: examination of the role of aluminum contamination. Saskatoon, Sk: 2004. Chris Arnold.

[24] Drongowski, RA; Coran, AG. An analysis of factors contributing to the development of total parenteral nutrition-induced cholestasis. *J Parenteral Enteral Nutr*, 1989, 13, 586–9.

[25] Postuma, R; Trevenen, CL. Liver disease in infants receiving total parenteral nutrition. *Pediatrics*, 1979, 63, 1 10-115.

[26] Dahms, BB; Halpin, Jr TC. Serial liver biopsies in parenteral nutrition associated cholestasis of early infancy. *Gastroenterology*, 1981, 81, 136-44.

[27] Kelly, D. Liver complications of pediatric parenteral nutrition-epidemiology. *Nutrition*, 1998, 14, 153–157.

[28] Mutanen, A; Lohi, J; Heikkila, P; Koivusalo, AI; Rintala, RJ; Pakarinen, MP. Persistent abnormal liver fibrosis after weaning off parenteral nutrition in pediatric intestinal failure. *Hepatology*, 2013, 58(2), 729-38.

[29] Costa, S; Maggio, L; Sindico, P; Cota, F; De, Carolis, MP; Romagnoli, C. Preterm small for gestational age infants are not at higher risk for parenteral nutrition–associated cholestasis. *J Pediatr*, 2010, 156, 575-9.

[30] Guglielmi, FW; Regano, N; Mazzuoli, S; Fregnan, S; Leogrande, G; Guglielmi, A; Merli, M; Pironi, L; Penco, JM; Francavilla, A. Cholestasis induced by total parenteral nutrition. *Clinics in Liver Disease*, 2008, 12(1), 97-110.

[31] Matory, JA. Jaundice. In: Hertz DE, editor. Care of the newborn: a handbook for primary care.1st ed. Philadelphia: Lippincott Williams and Wilkins, 2005.

[32] Balistreri, WF; Heubi, JE; Suchy, FJ. Immaturity of the enterohepatic circulation in early life: factors predisposing to "physiologic" maldigestion and cholestasis. *Journal of Pediatric Gastroenterology & Nutrition*, 1983, 2(2), 346-54.

[33] Hofmann, AF. Defective biliary secretion during total parenteral nutrition: probable mechanisms and possible solutions. *Journal of Pediatric Gastroenterology & Nutrition*, 1995, 20(4), 376-90.

[34] Rager, R; Finegold, MJ. Cholestasis in immature newborn infants: is parenteral alimentation responsible? *Journal of Pediatrics*, 1975, 86(2), 264-9.

[35] Tomer, G; Ananthanarayanan, M; Weymann, A; Balasubramanian, N; Suchy, FJ. Differential developmental regulation of rat liver canalicular membrane transporters Bsep and Mrp2. *Pediatr Res*, 2003, 53, 288–294.

[36] Chen, HL; Chen, HL; Liu, YJ; Feng, CH; Wu, CY; Shyu, MK; et al. Developmental expression of canalicular transporter genes in human liver. *J Hepatol*, 2005, 43, 472-477.

[37] Arrese, M; Ananthanarayanan, M. The bile salt export pump: molecular properties, function and regulation. *Pflugers Arch*, 2004, 449, 123–131.

[38] Kullak-Ublick, GA; Stieger, B; Meier, PJ. Enterohepatic bile salt transporters in normal physiology and liver disease. *Gastroenterology*, 2004, 126, 322–342.

[39] Alrefai1, WA; and, Gill, RK. Bile acid transporters: structure, function, regulation and pathophysiological implications. *Pharmaceutical Research*, 2007, 24(10), 1803-1823.

[40] Elferink, RO; Groen, AK. Genetic defects in hepatobiliary transport. *Biochim. Biophys. Acta.*, 2002, 1586, 129–145.

[41] Schmitt, M; Kubitz, R; Lizun, S; Wettstein, M; Haussinger, D. Regulation of the dynamic localization of the rat Bsep gene-encoded bile salt export pump by anisoosmolarity. *Hepatology*, 2001, 33, 509–518.

[42] Zollner, G; Fickert, P; Silbert, D; Fuchsbichler, A; Marschall, HU; Zatloukal, K; Denk, H; Trauner, M. Adaptive changes in hepatobiliary transporter expression in primary biliary cirrhosis. *J. Hepatol*, 2003, 38, 717–727.

[43] Wolters, H; Elzinga, BM; Baller, JF; Boverhof, R; Schwarz, M; Stieger, B; Verkade, HJ; Kuipers, F. Effects of bile salt flux variations on the expression of hepatic bile salt transporters in vivo in mice. *J. Hepatol*, 2002, 37, 556–563.

[44] Zollner, G; Fickert, P; Zenz, R; Fuchsbichler, A; Stumptner, C; Kenner, L; et al. Hepatobiliary transporter expression in percutaneous liver

biopsies of patients with cholestatic liver diseases. *Hepatology*, 2001, 33, 633–646.

[45] Li, J; Gong, YM; Wu, J; Wu, WJ; Cai, W. Anti-tumor necrosis factor-alpha monoclonal antibody alleviates parenteral nutrition-associated liver disease in mice. Jpen: *Journal of Parenteral & Enteral Nutrition*, 2012, 36(2), 219-25.

[46] González, MA; Roma, MG; Bernal, CA; Alvarez, ML; and, Carrillo, MC. Biliary secretory function in rats chronically intoxicated with aluminum. *Toxicol. Sci.*, 2004, 79, 189–195.

[47] Zelcer, N; van, de, Wetering, K; de, Waart, R; Scheffer, GL; Marschall, HU; Wielinga, PR; et al. Mice lacking Mrp3 (Abcc3) have normal bile salt transport, but altered hepatic transport of endogenous glucuronides. *J. Hepatol*, 2006, 44, 768–775.

[48] Oswald, M; Kullak-Ublick, A; Paumgartner, G; Beuers, U. Expression of hepatic transporters OATP-C and MRP2 in primary sclerosing cholangitis. *Liver*, 2001, 21, 247–253.

[49] Tazuke, Y; Kiristioglu, I; Heidelberger, KP; et al. Hepatic P-glycoprotein changes with total parenteral nutrition administration. *JPEN*, 2004, 28, 1–6.

[50] Kojima, H; Nies, AT; Konig, J; et al. Changes in the expression and localization of hepatocellular transporters and radixin in primary biliary cirrhosis. *J. Hepatol*, 2003, 39, 693–702.

[51] Shoda, J; Kano, M; Oda, K; Kamiya, J; Nimura, Y; Suzuki, H; et al. The expression levels of plasma membrane transporters in the cholestatic liver of patients undergoing biliary drainage and their association with the impairment of biliary secretory function. *Am J Gastroenterol*, 2001, 96, 3368–3378.

[52] Kojima, H; Sakurai, S; et al. The role of radixin in altered localization of canalicular conjugate export pump Mrp2 in cholestatic rat liver. *Hepatology Research*, 2008, 38, 202-210.

[53] Kojima, H; Sakurai, S; Uemura, M; Kitamura, K; Kanno, H; Nakai, Y; Fukui, H. Disturbed colocalization of multidrug resistance protein 2 and radixin in human cholestatic liver diseases. *Journal of Gastroenterology & Hepatology*, 2008, 23(7 Pt 2), e120-8.

[54] Kikuchi, S; Hata, M; Fukumoto, K; Yamane, Y; Matsui, T; Tamura, A; et al. Radixin deficiency causes conjugated hyperbilirubinemia with loss of Mrp2 from bile canalicular membranes. *Nature Genetics*, 2002, 31(3), 320-5.

[55] Ho, RH; Leake, BF; Roberts, RL; Lee, W; Kim, RB. Ethnicity-dependent polymorphism in Na+-taurocholate cotransporting polypeptide (SLC10A1) reveals a domain critical for bile acid substrate recognition. *J. Biol. Chem.*, 2004, 279, 7213–7222.

[56] Trauner, M; Arrese, M; Lee, H; Boyer, JL; Karpen, SJ. Endotoxin downregulates rat hepatic ntcp gene expression via decreased activity of critical transcription factors. *J. Clin. Invest.*, 1998, 101, 2092–2100.

[57] Hagenbuch, B; Meier, PJ. The superfamily of organic anion transporting polypeptides. *Biochim. Biophys. Acta*, 2003, 1609, 1–18.

[58] McClure, RJ; Newell, SJ. Randomised controlled trial of trophic feeding and gut motility. *Arch Dis Child Fetal Neonatal Ed.*, 1999, 80(1), F54-8.

[59] Omata, J; Fukatsu, K; Murakoshi, S; Noguchi, M; Miyazaki, H; Moriya, T; et al. Enteral refeeding rapidly restores PN-induced reduction of hepatic mononuclear cell number through recovery of small intestine and portal vein blood flows. Jpen: *Journal of Parenteral & Enteral Nutrition*, 2009, 33(6), 618-25.

[60] Lambert, JR; Thomas, SM. Metronidazole prevention of serum liver enzyme abnormalities during total parenteral nutrition. Jpen: *Journal of Parenteral & Enteral Nutrition*, 1985, 9(4), 501-3.

[61] Trauner, M; Fickert, P; Stauber, RE. Inflammation-induced cholestasis. *J Gastroenterol Hepatol*, 1999, 14, 946-59.

[62] Fuchs, M; Sanyal, AJ. Sepsis and cholestasis. *Clinics in Liver Disease*, 2008, 12(1), 151-72, ix.

[63] El, Kasmi, KC; Anderson, AL; Devereaux, MW; Fillon, SA; Harris, JK; Lovell, MA; Finegold, MJ; Sokol, RJ. Toll-like receptor 4-dependent Kupffer cell activation and liver injury in a novel mouse model of parenteral nutrition and intestinal injury. *Hepatology*, 2012, 55(5), 1518-28.

[64] Burjonrappa, SC; Miller, M. Role of trace elements in parenteral nutrition support of the surgical neonate. *Journal of Pediatric Surgery*, 2012, 47(4), 760-71.

[65] Fell, JM; Reynolds, AP; Meadows, N; Khan, K; Long, SG; Quaghebeur, G; Taylor, WJ; Milla, PJ. Manganese toxicity in children receiving long-term parenteral nutrition. *Lancet*, 1996, 347(9010), 1218-21.

[66] Reynolds, AP; Kiely, E; Meadows N. Manganese in long term paediatric parenteral nutrition. *Arch Dis Child*, 1994, 71(6), 527-8.

[67] Hardy, G. Manganese in parenteral nutrition: who, when, and why should we supplement? *Gastroenterology*, 2009, 137(5 Suppl), S29-35.

[68] Slicker, J; Vermilyea, S. Pediatric parenteral nutrition: putting the microscope on macronutrients and micronutrients. [Erratum appears in Nutr Clin Pract. 2009, 24(5), 655 Note: Dosage error in article text] *Nutrition in Clinical Practice*, 2009, 24(4), 481-6.

[69] Koletzko, B; Agostoni, C; Ball, P; Carnielli, V; Chaloner, C; Clayton, J; et al. ESPEN/ESPGHAN Guidelines on paediatric parenteral nutrition. *Journal of Pediatric Gastroenterology and Nutrition*, 2005, 41, S1-S87.

[70] Blaszyk, H; Wild, PJ; Oliveira, A; et al. Hepatic copper in patients receiving long-term total parenteral nutrition. *J Clin Gastroenterol*, 2005, 39(4), 318-20.

[71] Poole, RL; Schiff, L; Hintz, SR; Wong, A; Mackenzie, N; Kerner, JA Jr. Aluminum content of parenteral nutrition in neonates: measured versus calculated levels. *J Pediatr Gastroenterol Nutr*, 2010, 50, 208-11.

[72] Gura, KM. Aluminum contamination in products used in parenteral nutrition: has anything changed? *Nutrition*, 2010, 26, 585-94.

[73] Federal Register. Aluminum in large and small volume parenterals used in total parenteral nutrition. *Fed Regist*, 2011, 21, 89-90.

[74] ASCN/ A.S.P.E.N. Working Group on Standards for Aluminum Content of Parenteral Nutrition Solutions. Parenteral drug products containing aluminum as an ingredient or a contaminant: Response to Food and Drug Administration notice of intent and request for information. *JPEN*, 1991, 15(2).

[75] Wier, HA; Kuhn, RJ. Aluminum toxicity in neonatal parenteral nutrition: what can we do? *Annals of Pharmacotherapy*, 2012, 46(1), 137-40.

[76] Smith, BS; Kothari, H; Hayes, BD; et al. Effect of additive selection on calculated aluminum content of parenteral nutrient solutions. *Am J Health Syst Pharm*, 2007, 64, 730-9.

[77] Robinson, DT; Steinhorn, RH. Pre-term neonate with intestinal failure, feeding issues. *Pediatric Annals*, 2011, 40(8), 404-6.

[78] Alemmari, A; Miller, GG; Arnold, CJ; Zello, GA. Parenteral aluminum induces liver injury in a newborn piglet model. *J Pediatr Surg*, 2011, 46(5), 883-7.

[79] Alemmari, A; Miller, GG; Bertolo, RF; Dinesh, C; Brunton, JA; Arnold, CJ; Zello, GA. Reduced aluminum contamination decreases parenteral nutrition associated liver injury. *Journal of Pediatric Surgery*, 2012, 47(5), 889-94.

[80] Arnold, CJ; Miller, GG; Zello, GA. Parenteral nutrition-associated cholestasis in neonates; the role of aluminum. *Nutr Rev*, 2003, 61(9), 306-10.

[81] Klein, G; Berquist, W; Ament, M; Coburn, J; Miller, N; Alfrey, A. Hepatic aluminum accumulation in children on total parenteral nutrition. *J Pediatr Gastroenterol Nutr*, 1984, 3, 740–743.
[82] Klein, G; Heyman, M; Lee, T; et al. Aluminum-associated hepatobiliary dysfunction in rats: relationships to dosage and duration of exposure. *Pediatr Res*, 1988, 23, 275–278.
[83] Demircan, M; Ergun, O; Coker, C; et al. Aluminum in total parenteral nutrition solutions produces portal inflammation in rats. *J Pediat Gastroenterol Nutr*, 1998, 26, 274–278
[84] Bertholf, RL; Herman, MM; Savory, J; et al. A long-term intravenous model of aluminum maltol toxicity in rabbits: tissue distribution, hepatic, renal and neuronal cytoskeletal changes associated with systemic exposure. *Toxicol. Appl. Pharmacol*, 1989, 98, 58-74.
[85] Gonzalez, MA; Alvarez, ML; Pisani, GB; et al. Involvement of oxidative stress in the impairment in biliary secretory function induced by intraperitoneal administration of aluminum to rats. *Biol Trace Elem Res*, 2007, 116, 329–348.
[86] UK Medicines and Healthcare Regulatory Agency. Calcium gluconate injection in small-volume glass containers: new contraindications due to aluminum exposure risk. *MHRA: Drug Safety Update*, 2010 August, 4(1), A2.
[87] Pharmaceutical Partners of Canada Inc. Calcium gluconate injection 10% - important information concerning the presence of aluminum - for health professionals [Internet]. Ottawa, Ont: Health Canada; 2011 [Updated: 2013-03, Accessed: 2013-04]. Available from: http://www.healthycanadians.gc.ca/recall-alert-rappel-avis/index-eng.php
[88] Pharmaceutical Partners of Canada Inc. Calcium gluconate injection, USP 10% [Package insert]. Richmond Hill, On: Pharmaceutical Partners of Canada Inc, 2008. [Accessed; 2013-04]. Available from: http://ppcdrugs.com/en/files/2012/09/EN_WebInsert_CalcGluc.pdf
[89] Vileisis, RA; Inwood, RJ; Hunt, CE. Prospective controlled study of parenteral nutrition–associated cholestatic jaundice: effect of protein intake. *J Pediatr*, 1980, 96(5), 893-7.
[90] Blau, J; Sridhar, S; Mathieson, S; et al. Effects of protein/nonprotein caloric intake on parenteral nutrition associated cholestasis in premature infants weighing 600-1000 grams. *JPEN J Parenter Enteral Nutr*, 2007, 31(6), 487-90.
[91] Clark, RH; Chace, DH; Spitzer, AR; et al. Effects of two different doses of amino acid supplementation on growth and blood amino acid levels in

premature neonates admitted to the neonatal intensive care unit: a randomized, controlled trial. *Pediatrics*, 2007, 120(6), 1286-96.

[92] Meguid, MM; Akahoshi, MP; Jeffers, S; Hayashi, RJ; Hammond, WG. Amelioration of metabolic complications of conventional total parenteral nutrition. A prospective randomized study. *Archives of Surgery*, 1984, 119(11), 1294-8.

[93] Wagner, WH; Lowry, AC; Silberman, H. Similar liver function abnormalities occur in patients receiving glucose-based and lipid-based parenteral nutrition. *American Journal of Gastroenterology*, 1983, 78(4), 199-202.

[94] Iyer, KR; Spitz, L; Clayton, P. BAPS prize lecture: new insight into mechanisms of parenteral nutrition–associated cholestasis: role of plant sterols. British Association of Paediatric Surgeons. *J Pediatr Surg*, 1998, 33(1), 1-6.

[95] Bindl, L; Lutjohann, D; Buderus, S; Lentze, MJ; v, Bergmann, K. High plasma levels of phytosterols in patients on parenteral nutrition: a marker of liver dysfunction. *Journal of Pediatric Gastroenterology & Nutrition*, 2000, 31(3), 313-6.

[96] Park, KT; Nespor, C; Kerner, J, Jr. The use of Omegaven in treating parenteral nutrition-associated liver disease. *Journal of Perinatology*, 2011, 31 Suppl 1, S57-60.

[97] Kurvinen, A; Nissinen, MJ; Gylling, H; Miettinen, TA; Lampela, H; Koivusalo, AI; Rintala, RJ; Pakarinen, MP. Effects of long-term parenteral nutrition on serum lipids, plant sterols, cholesterol metabolism, and liver histology in pediatric intestinal failure. *Journal of Pediatric Gastroenterology & Nutrition*, 2011, 53(4), 440-6.

[98] Carter, BA; Taylor, OA; Prendergast, DR; et al. Stigmasterol, a soy lipid-derived phytosterol, is an antagonist of the bile acid nuclear receptor FXR. *Pediatr Res*, 2007, 62, 301-306.

[99] Shefer, S; Salen, G; Nguyen, L; Batta, AK; Packing, V; Tint, GS; Hauser, S. Competitive inhibition of bile acid synthesis by endogenous cholestanol and sitosterol in sitosterolemia with xanthomatosis: effect on cholesterol 7 alpha-hydroxylase. *J Clin Invest*, 1988, 82, 1833–9.

[100] Clayton, PT; Whitfield, P; Iyer, K. The role of phytosterols in the pathogenesis of liver complications of pediatric parenteral nutrition. *Nutrition*, 1998, 14, 158-64.

[101] Savini, S; D'Ascenzo, R; Biagetti, C; Serpentini, G; Pompilio, A; Bartoli, A; Cogo, PE; Carnielli, VP. The effect of 5 intravenous lipid emulsions on plasma phytosterols in preterm infants receiving parenteral

nutrition: a randomized clinical trial. *American Journal of Clinical Nutrition*, 2013, 98(2), 312-8.

[102] Gura, KM; Lee, S; Valim, C; et al. Safety and efficacy of a fish oil-based fat emulsion in the treatment of parenteral nutrition–associated liver disease. *Pediatrics*, 2008, 121, e678-e686.

[103] Cober, MP; Teitelbaum, DH. Prevention of parenteral nutrition–associated liver disease: lipid minimization. *Curr Opin Organ Transplant*, 2010, 15(3), 330-3.

[104] Cowan, E; Nandivada, P; Puder, M. Fish oil-based lipid emulsion in the treatment of parenteral nutrition-associated liver disease. *Current Opinion in Pediatrics*, 2013, 25(2), 193-200.

[105] Le, HD; Meisel, JA; de, Meijer, VE; et al. The essentiality of arachidonic acid and docosahexaenoic acid. *Prostaglandins Leukot Essent Fatty Acids*, 2009, 81(2-3), 165-70.

[106] Klek, S; Chambrier, C; Singer, P; Rubin, M; Bowling, T; Staun, M; et al. Four-week parenteral nutrition using a third generation lipid emulsion (SMOFlipid)--a double-blind, randomised, multicentre study in adults. *Clinical Nutrition*, 2013, 32(2), 224-31.

[107] Goulet, O; Antebi, H; Wolf, C; et al. A new intravenous fat emulsion containing soybean oil, medium-chain triglycerides, olive oil, and fish oil; a single-center, double-blind randomized study on efficacy and safety in pediatric patients receiving home parenteral nutrition. *JPEN J Parenter Enteral Nutr*, 2010, 34(5), 485-95.

[108] Sant'Anna, AM; Altamimi, E; Clause, RF; Saab, J; Mileski, H; Cameron, B; Fitzgerald, P; Sant'Anna, GM. Implementation of a multidisciplinary team approach and fish oil emulsion administration in the management of infants with short bowel syndrome and parenteral nutrition-associated liver disease. *Canadian Journal of Gastroenterology*, 2012, 26(5), 277-80.

[109] Javid, PJ; Collier, S; Richardson, D; Iglesias, J; Gura, K; Lo, C; et al. The role of enteral nutrition in the reversal of parenteral nutrition–associated liver dysfunction in infants. *J Pediatr Surg*, 2005, 40, 1015-8.

[110] Meehan, JJ; Georgeson, KE. Prevention of liver failure in parenteral nutrition–dependent children with short bowel syndrome. *J Pediatr Surg*, 1997, 132, 473-5.

[111] De, Curtis, M; Rigo, J. The nutrition of preterm infants. *Early Human Development*, 2012, 88 Suppl 1, S5-7.

[112] Salvador, A; Janeczko, M; Porat, R; Sekhon, R; Moewes, A; Schutzman, D. Randomized controlled trial of early parenteral nutrition cycling to

prevent cholestasis in very low birth weight infants. *Journal of Pediatrics*, 2012, 161(2), 229-33.e1.

[113] Jensen, AR; Goldin, AB; Koopmeiners, JS; Stevens, J; Waldhausen, JHT; Kim, SS. The association of cyclic parenteral nutrition and decreased cholestasis in patients with gastroschisis. *J Pediatr Surg*, 2009, 44, 183-9.

[114] Beuers, U. Drug insight: mechanisms and sites of action of ursodeoxycholic acid in cholestasis. *Nat Clin Pract Gastroenterol Hepatol*, 2006, 3, 318-328.

[115] Spagnuolo, MI; Iorio, R; Vegnente, A; et al. Ursodeoxycholic acid for treatment of cholestasis in children on long-term total parenteral nutrition: a pilot study. *Gastroenterology*, 1996, 111(3), 716-9.

[116] De, Marco, G; Sordino, D; Bruzzese, E; et al. Early treatment with ursodeoxycholic acid for cholestasis in children on parenteral nutrition because of primary intestinal failure. *Aliment Pharmacol Ther*, 2006, 24, 387-394.

[117] Heubi, JE; Wiechmann, DA; Creutzinger, V; et al. Tauroursodeoxycholic acid (TUDCA) in the prevention of total parenteral nutrition–associated liver disease. *J Pediatr*, 2002, 141, 237-242.

[118] Teitelbaum, DH; Tracy, TF, Jr; Aouthmany, MM; Llanos, A; Brown, MB; Yu, S; et al. Use of cholecystokinin-octapeptide for the prevention of parenteral nutrition-associated cholestasis. *Pediatrics*, 2005, 115(5), 1332-40.

[119] Jain, AK; Stoll, B; Burrin, DG; Holst, JJ; Moore, DD. Enteral bile acid treatment improves parenteral nutrition-related liver disease and intestinal mucosal atrophy in neonatal pigs. *American Journal of Physiology - Gastrointestinal & Liver Physiology*, 2012, 302(2), G218-24.

[120] Tsai, S; Strouse, PJ; Drongowski, RA; et al. Failure of cholecystokinin octapeptide to prevent TPN-associated gallstone disease. *J Pediatr Surg*, 2005, 40(1), 263-7.

[121] Spencer, AU; Yu, S; Tracy, TF; et al. Parenteral nutrition–associated cholestasis in neonates: multivariate analysis of the potential protective effect of taurine. *JPEN J Parenter Enteral Nutr*, 2005, 29(5), 337-43

[122] Zaman, N; Tam, YK; Jewell, LD; Coutts, RT. Effects of taurine supplementation in parenteral nutrition-associated hepatosteatosis and lidocaine metabolism. A study using isolated rat liver perfusion. *Drug Metabolism & Disposition*, 1996, 24(5), 534-41.

[123] Carter, RJ; Shulman, BA. Mechanism of disease: update on the molecular etiology and fundamentals of parenteral nutrition associated cholestasis. *Nat Clin Pract Gastroenterol Hepatol*, 2007, 4, 277–287.

[124] Wu, J; Wang, X; Cai, W; Hong, L; Tang, Q. Bifidobacterium adolescentis supplementation ameliorates parenteral nutrition-induced liver injury in infant rabbits. *Digestive Diseases & Sciences*, 2010, 55(10), 2814-20.

[125] Tillman, EM. Review and clinical update on parenteral nutrition-associated liver disease. *Nutrition in Clinical Practice*, 2013, 28(1), 30-9.

[126] Fallon, EM; Le, HD; Puder, M. Prevention of parenteral nutrition-associated liver disease: role of omega-3 fish oil. *Current Opinion in Organ Transplantation*, 2010, 15(3), 334-40.

[127] Oshita, M; Takehara, H; Yamaguchi, M; et al. Significance of administration of fat emulsion: hepatic changes in infant rats receiving total parenteral nutrition with and without fat. *Clin Nutr*, 2004, 23(5), 1060-8.

[128] Sanchez, SE; Braun, LP; Mercer, LD; Sherrill, M; Stevens, J; Javid, PJ. The effect of lipid restriction on the prevention of parenteral nutrition-associated cholestasis in surgical infants. *Journal of Pediatric Surgery*, 2013, 48(3), 573-8.

[129] Gura, KM; Duggan, CP; Collier, SB; Jennings, RW; Folkman, J; Bistrian, BR; Puder, M. Reversal of parenteral nutrition-associated liver disease in two infants with short bowel syndrome using parenteral fish oil: implications for future management. *Pediatrics*, 2006, 118(1), e197-201.

[130] de, Meijer, VE; Le, HD; Meisel, JA; et al. Parenteral fish oil as monotherapy prevents essential fatty acid deficiency in parenteral nutrition-dependent patients. *J Pediatr Gastroenterol Nutr*, 2010, 50(2), 212-8.

[131] Premkumar, MH; Carter, BA; Hawthorne, KM; King, K; Abrams, SA. High rates of resolution of cholestasis in parenteral nutrition-associated liver disease with fish oil-based lipid emulsion monotherapy. *Journal of Pediatrics*, 2013, 162(4), 793-798.e1.

[132] Puder, M; Valim, C; Meisel, JA; Le, HD; de, Meijer, VE; Robinson, EM; et al. Parenteral fish oil improves outcomes in patients with parenteral nutrition-associated liver injury. *Ann Surg*, 2009, 250, 395-402.

[133] Piper, SN; Schade, I; Beschmann, RB; Maleck, WH; Boldt, J; Rohm, KD. Hepatocellular integrity after parenteral nutrition: comparison of a fish-oil-containing lipid emulsion with an olive-soybean oil-based lipid emulsion. *European Journal of Anaesthesiology*, 2009, 26, 1076-1082.

[134] Vanel, VW; Seider, DL; Allen, P; et al. A.S.P.E.N. Position Paper: Clinical Role for Alternative Intravenous Fat Emulsions. *Nutrition in Clinical Practice*, 2012, 27(2), 150-192.

[135] Thatch, KA; Katz, MS; Haber, MM; Schwartz, MZ. Growth factor modulation of hepatic inflammation: a novel approach to the management of total parenteral nutrition-associated liver disease. *Journal of Pediatric Surgery*, 2010, 45(1), 89-94.

[136] Demircan, M; Uguralp, S; Mutus, M; Gurer, EI; Atik, E; Turhan, F; Gursoy, MH. The effects of acetylsalicylic acid, interferon-alpha, and vitamin E on prevention of parenteral nutrition-associated cholestasis: an experimental study. *Journal of Pediatric Gastroenterology & Nutrition*, 1999, 28(3), 291-5.

In: Parenteral Nutrition
Editor: Shana Lelio

ISBN: 978-1-63321-112-4

Chapter 5

Current Management of Parenteral Nutrition-Associated Liver Disease in Adults

Yousheng Li*, M.D., Ph.D.
Director, Intestinal Rehabilitation and Transplantation Center,
Jinling Hospital, Nanjing University School of Medicine,
Nanjing, China

Abstract

Parenteral nutrition-associated liver disease (PNALD) has been common in patients who require long-term parenteral nutrition (PN), it occurs in 15%-40% of adults receiving home PN and 40%-60% of infants receiving long-term PN for intestinal failure (IF). Clinical diagnosis of PNALD includes biochemical markers for liver disease, such as aspartate aminotransferase (AST), alanine aminotransferase (ALT), total bilirubin (TB), direct bilirubin (DB), and ruling out all other potential causes of liver disease. Meanwhile, liver biopsy is needed to definitively diagnose PNALD. The pathogenesis of PNALD is multifactorial and remains unclear. Risk factors include disruption of the enterohepatic circulation of bile acids, intestinal stasis with subsequent bacterial overgrowth, bile sludging with subsequent bile duct obstruction, early and/or recurrent

* E-mail: liys@medmail.com.cn.

central venous catheter-related sepsis, and nutrient deficiency or excess. There is no specific treatment. Management strategies for its prevention and treatment depend on an understanding of many risk factors, and in general include consideration of early enteral feeding, the use of specialized lipid emulsions such as fish oil emulsions, and isolated small intestinal or combined liver-intestinal transplantation.

Keywords: Parenteral nutrition-associated liver disease; parenteral nutrition; sepsis; emulsions; fish oil; isolated small intestinal transplantation; combined liver-intestinal transplantation

1. Introduction

Mainstreaming of long-term PN has profoundly impacted the prognosis and quality of lives of individuals with IF from congenital abnormalities or extensive gastrointestinal surgery. Although PN is life-saving, its long-term use is associated with severe adverse effects, including septic infection, metabolic imbalance and hepatobiliary dysfunction. The hepatobiliary complications of PN are now well recognized as PNALD, which is associated with increased morbidity and mortality. PNALD is also referred to as PN-associated cholestasis (PNAC), PN-associated liver injury (PNALI), or, more recently, intestinal failure-associated liver disease (IFALD). Because PNALD typically improves with the advancement of enteral nutrition (EN) and the discontinuation of PN, and IF encompasses patients who necessitate specialized nutrition support as EN and/or PN, I have chosen to use PNALD throughout this article.

PNALD is usually associated with prolonged PN administration (> 2 weeks) and is characterized by cholestasis and hepatic dysfunction, including biochemical and histological alterations ranging from mild elevation of hepatic transaminases to steatosis, cirrhosis, and end-stage liver failure. PNALD has been common in both adults and infants who require long-term PN, it is estimated to be approximately 40%-60% in infants and up to 85% in neonates who are receiving long-term PN for IF and 15%-40% in adults who are receiving home PN. Clinical diagnosis of PNALD includes biochemical markers for liver disease, such as AST, ALT, TB, DB, and ruling out all other potential causes of liver disease. Although liver biopsy is needed to definitively diagnose PNALD, because of the invasive nature of biopsy, many centers will not perform diagnostic liver biopsies and consider DB > 2 or 3 mg/dL in the absence of any other liver etiology reflective of PNALD.

PNALD is one of the most devastating complications affecting patients receiving PN. The etiology of PNALD is not well understood and is likely multifactorial. The purpose of this review is to provide some historical prospective on PNALD but focusing more on recent literature pertaining to the treatment and etiology of PNALD.

2. Risk Factors

Despite the widespread use of PN in clinical practice for more than 30 years, and its well-documented association with cholestatic liver disease, the precise etiology of PNALD remains a mystery. However, the pathogenesis of PNALD in adults appears to be multifactorial, suggested theories include disruption of the enterohepatic circulation of bile acids, intestinal stasis with subsequent bacterial overgrowth, bile sludging with subsequent bile duct obstruction, early and/or recurrent central venous catheter-related sepsis, and nutrient deficiency or excess (Figure 1).

2.1. Nutrient Deficiency

Deficiency of some micronutrients such as choline, taurine, chromium, aluminum, oxidants and lipids may be involved in the pathogenesis of PNALD.

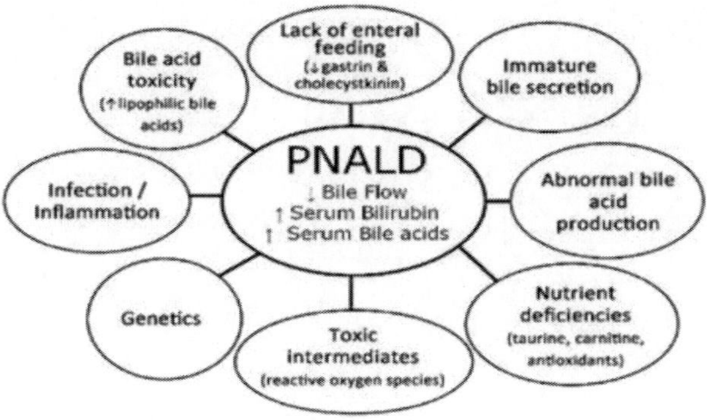

Figure 1. Multifactorial pathophysiology associated with PNALD.

2.1.1. Choline

Choline, one of the pathway products of choline synthesis, is a nutrient found in many foods but is not considered essential because of endogenous synthesis is possible from methionine contained in the crystalline amino acid solution (Figure 2), it is low in > 90% of the patients who require long-term total PN (TPN).

The biosynthesis of choline may be inadequate when methionine is given parenterally than when it enters the liver via the portal vein. Fortunately, hepatic steatosis that resulted from choline deficiency may be reversed by the addition of choline to PN solutions. A group of 15 adult patients receiving long-term PN with hepatic steatosis confirmed by CT were randomized to receive their usual PN formulation, or one supplemented with 2 g choline chloride daily for 24 weeks. Only 9 patients completed the study, but steatosis resolved in the 4 patients who received choline and none of the 5 patients who did not receive choline as determined by liver/spleen CT scanning. In addition, 2 of the choline-supplemented patients who returned for follow-up 10 weeks after choline had been discontinued had recurrence of steatosis. In a pediatric population, 21 children receiving long-term PN were compared with 31 normal controls. The mean plasma free choline concentrations were significantly lower in the long-term PN patients than the control group and showed a steady and significant decline with increased age. In addition, a significant negative correlation was shown between plasma free choline concentration and serum hepatic aminotransferase concentrations.

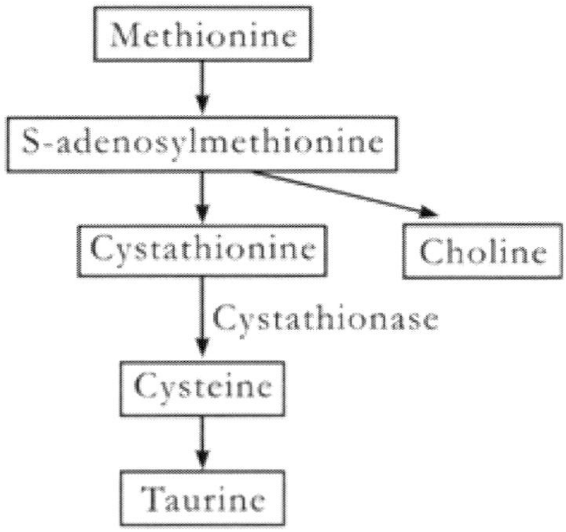

Figure 2. A schematic diagram of the hepatic transsulfuration pathway from methionine to taurine (some intermediates are omitted for clarity).

Additional studies are under way to further evaluate the role of choline in the prevention and treatment of PNALD. At present, there is no injectable choline preparation commercially available.

2.1.2. Taurine

Deficiency of taurine, another product of the hepatic transsulfuration pathway, could play a role in the development of PNALD in neonates, this deficiency leads to the inability to form taurine-conjugated bile acids efficiently and, unfortunately, favors the formation of hydrophobic and toxic glycine-conjugated bile acids. In older infants and adults, taurine is synthesized from methionine, but is diminished owing to cystathionase deficiency in premature infants.

Cystathionase is the rate-limiting enzyme in the formation of cysteine from cystathionine, an intermediate in the metabolism from methionine to taurine (Figure 2). In a large prospective multicenter study conducted between 1996 and 2001, the presence or absence of taurine in PN formulations was analyzed by multivariate analysis.

The choice of taurine supplementation in these patients was based on the individual hospital formulary that provided either the standardized adult crystalline amino acid solution or the specialized neonatal amino acid solution supplemented with taurine.

2.2. Nutrient Excess

2.2.1. Caloric Loads

Caloric loads in PN, in the form of either dextrose or amino acids, have been associated with hepatic pathological and biochemical changes. For example, in both animals and humans, caloric excess is associated with elevated transaminase levels and hepatic steatosis. In addition, amino acid infusions have been associated with cholestatic liver disease in humans and animals.

Vileisis et al. had demonstrated that premature infants who received daily amino acids of 3.6 g/kg had a more rapid rise in bilirubin levels than those who received 2.5 g/kg daily. Our animal investigation showed that the incidence of PNALD in rats received high-energy TPN (260 kcal/kg/d of non-protein energy) was higher than that in rats received low-energy TPN (160 kcal/kg/d).

2.2.2. Dextrose

Dextrose-based PN formulations that contain little or no fat have been implicated in the development of steatosis. Not only do excess carbohydrates deposit in the liver as fat, but a dextrose-based PN formulation may result in the development of essential fatty acid deficiency (EFAD). EFAD may lead to impaired lipoprotein formation and triglyceride secretion and result in steatosis.

Providing a balanced dextrose and fat source of calories appears to decrease the incidence of steatosis, possibly by decreasing hepatic triglyceride uptake, and promoting fatty acid oxidation. Now that dextrose-based PN formulations have essentially been replaced with a more balanced dextrose-fat formulation and less overall calories are provided than previously estimated, the incidence of steatosis has decreased. Our experimental studies showed that steatosis occurred when dextrose was given solely as non-protein calorie. Therefore, it is recommended that a balanced PN formulation provide 70%-85% of non-protein calories as carbohydrate and 15%-30% as fat. In addition, carbohydrate content should not exceed 7 g/kg/d in adults.

2.2.3. Amino Acids

Early sources of amino acids for parenteral use included protein hydrolysates that had significant amounts of aluminum contamination. Animal studies have suggested that high levels of aluminum contamination may lead to the development of cholestasis. Five pediatric patients who developed cholestasis and were receiving PN that contained casein hydrolysate as the protein source demonstrated markedly elevated hepatic aluminum content on biopsy. However, the replacement of protein hydrolysates with crystalline amino acids has significantly reduced the overall aluminum contamination in PN formulations and is no longer considered a significant risk factor for the development of liver complications.

2.2.4. Lipids

Intravenous lipid emulsions are an essential component of PN regimens, representing a major source of energy and essential fatty acids (FAs). Intralipid, the first commercially available lipid emulsion, is based on soybean oil and characterized by a high content of essential long-chain poly-unsaturated fatty acids (LC-PUFA), linoleic (LA, ω-6, 52%-54%) and α-linolenic (ALA, ω-3, 7%-9%) acid. However, because of the high supply of LA, alternative lipid emulsions are developed by partially replacing soybean oil with other lipids such as medium-chain triglycerides (MCT), olive oil.

MCT are rapidly cleared from the bloodstream and are less susceptible to lipid peroxidation than PUFA. Olive oil is rich in the monounsaturated fatty acid (MUFA). Linoleic acid is less prone to lipid peroxidation than PUFA due to its chemical structure. The vegetable oil-based lipid emulsions such as soybean, safflower oils contain high concentrations of ω-6 fatty acids (ω-6 PUFAs) and phytosterols, which are associated with impaired biliary secretion and hypothesized to contribute to liver injury. The composition of the lipids in these emulsions is shown in Table 1.

Fish oil contains ω-3 PUFAs, eicosapentaenoic acid (EPA) and docosahexaenoic acid (DHA). Down-stream products of ω-6 PUFAs are the pro-inflammatory four-series leukotrienes (leukotriene B4, C4, E4), the two-series prostaglandins (prostaglandin E2, prostacyclin I2), and thromboxane A2. These eicosanoids are mediated by cyclooxygenase and 5-lipooxy-genase and thought to promote liver inflammation (Figure 3). Due to their favourable immunomodulatory and anti-inflammatory properties, provision of EPA and DHA has been considered to be of benefit in patients at risk of inflammation and sepsis.

Table 1. Comparison and characteristics of parenteral lipid emulsions (100 g fat/L)

Product Manufacturer	Intralipid Baxter Healthcare/Fresenius Kabi	Liposyn II Hospira	ClinOleic Baxter Healthcare/ Parenteral S.A.	SMOF lipid Fresenius Kabi	Omegaven Fresenius Kabi
Oil source (g)					
Soybean	10	5	2	3	0
Safflower	0	5	0	0	0
MCT	0	0	0	3	0
Olive oil	0	0	8	2.5	0
α-Tocopherol (mg/l)	38	NR	32	200	150–296
Phytosterols (mg/l)	348±33	383	327±8	47.6	0
Fat composition (g)					
Linoleic	5.0	6.5	0.9	2.9	0.1–0.7
α-Linolenic	0.9	0.4	0.1	0.3	<0.2
EPA	0	0	0	0.3	1.28–2.82
DHA	0	0	0	0.05	1.44–3.09
Oleic	2.6	1.8	2.8	2.8	0.6–1.3
Palmitic	1.0	0.9	0.7	0.9	0.25–1
Stearic	0.35	0.34	0.2	0.3	0.05–0.2
Arachidonic	0	0	0.03	0.05	0.1–0.4

DHA, docosahexaenoic acid; EPA, eicosapentaenoic acid; MCT, medium chain triglyceride; NR, not reported.

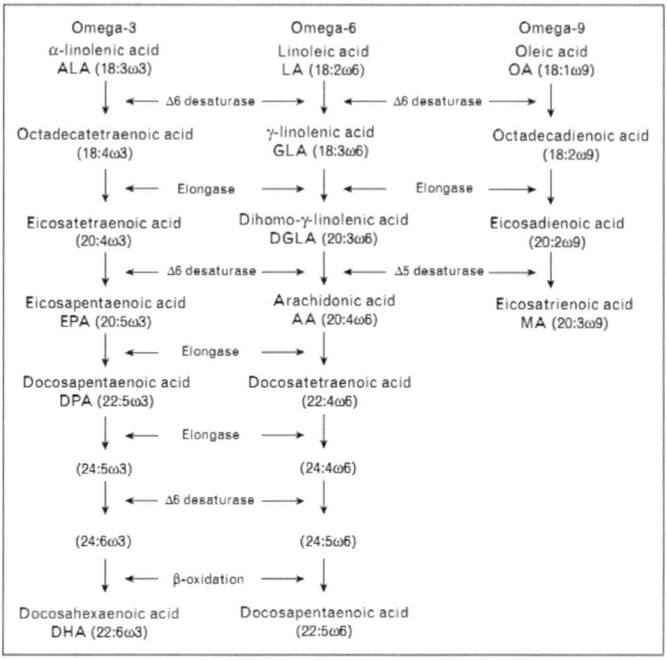

Figure 3. Role of ω-3 PUFAs and ω-6 PUFAs in inflammation.

There are various concerns regarding the role of lipids in the development of liver complications, including the fat source, the phytosterol content, and the dose. The source of lipids may play a role in risk of developing liver complications. Two characteristics of lipid emulsions have been implicated as etiologic factors in this process: phytosterol content and the pro-inflammatory nature of ω-6 PUFAs.

2.2.5. Phytosterols

Phytosterols, naturally occurring in plants, are plant-derived steroid alcohols. They are the component of the cell membrane, the role which is played by cholesterol in mammalian systems. Formulations of lipid emulsions contain high levels of phytosterols, and animal data suggested that these agents may lead to impaired bile drainage and hepatobiliary dysfunction. In a mammalian animal model, the neonatal piglets were given sterol and measured phytosterol accumulation in the serum, liver, and bile and compared them to non-exposed piglets. The sterol-treated piglets had significantly higher serum bile acid levels and lower maximal bile acid accumulation. Furthermore, phytosterols caused a significant inhibition of secretory functions in isolated rat hepatocyte couplets. Formulations of lipid emulsions do contain a reversed ratio of phytosterols to cholesterol when compared with the normal human diet. Kurvinen et al. recently demonstrated a positive correlation between the concentration of serum phytosterols and the degree of liver disease. PNALD is defined as a level of above 1.5 times the upper limit of normal of at least two of three of the following: DB > 35 mmol/L, gamma-glutamyl transpeptidase (GGT) > 75 U/L, and ALT > 65 U/L. Patients who have higher levels of ALT and DB also have higher levels of phytosterols in their serum. The mechanism of phytosterols induced liver injury is not clear. It has been postulated that Farnesoid X Receptor (FXR) has the key factor. FXR is a bile acid ligand-activated nuclear receptor that, once activated, suppresses 7-α-hydroxylase, the rate-limiting enzyme in bile acid synthesis. Thus, FXR regulates bile acid homeostasis by providing a route of negative feedback when bile acids are already elevated in the body. When FXR is inhibited, as is the case with phytosterols, bile acid homeostasis is disrupted, leading to liver injury and cholestasis.

2.2.6. Inflammatory Mediators

Although both ω-6 PUFAs and ω-3 PUFAs serve as lipid precursors for the synthesis of inflammatory mediators, the potency of the inflammatory response is highly dependent on the type of mediator produced. ω-6 PUFAs metabolism predominantly results in the production of the 2-series prostaglandins and thromboxanes and the 4-series leukotrienes, including leukotriene B4 (Figure 3). These mediators result in the release of pro-inflammatory cytokines such as IL-6, initiating leukocyte chemotaxis, vasodilation, and the stimulation of pain pathways. Dominance of these pro-inflammatory mediators has been implicated in the pathogenesis of PNALD. It should be noted, however, that ω-6 PUFAs also serve as a source of anti-inflammatory mediators, with production of epoxyeicosatrienoic acids when metabolized by cytochrome P450 epoxygenases. In addition, ω-6 PUFAs-derived α-linolenic acid serves as a precursor for the less pro-inflammatory 1-series prostaglandins. However, epoxyeicosatrienoic acids and α-linolenic acid have not been investigated in PNALD. Alternatively, ω-3 PUFAs lead to the production of the 3-series prostaglandins and thromboxanes and the 5-series leukotrienes (Figure 3). Compared with the ω-6 PUFAs-derived eicosanoids, these mediators are less potent in their stimulation of pro-inflammatory pathways and in some cases have anti-inflammatory effects. Soybean-based lipid emulsions are rich in ω-6 PUFAs, which have been shown to promote hepatocyte damage or induce hepatocyte apoptosis through a pro-inflammatory mechanism.

2.2.7. Lipid Dosing

Lipid emulsions are recommended to be administered at a dose less than 2.5 g/kg/d. However, dosing at more than 1 g/kg/d has been associated with the development of PNALD, whereas dosing at 1 g/kg/d or less has been shown effective in preventing PNALD. In humans, biochemical changes associated with EFAD can occur in as little as a few days in infants and within several weeks in older children and adults. EFAD typically occurs when less than 1%-2% of total calories are provided from essential fatty acids. As adults have a larger storage of essential fatty acids, symptoms of EFAD such as dry skin, alopecia, and dermatitis rarely occur. Premature infants, however, require at least 4% of total calories from essential fatty acids to prevent growth retardation and inadequate brain development. The enzymatic pathways of the neonate and premature infant are not adequately developed and do not efficiently convert ALA and linoleic acid to the active moieties DHA and arachidonic acid.

2.3. Sepsis

Septic events are a major risk factor in the development of PNALD in patients with IF. Diamond et al found that each septic episode was associated with a 3.2-fold increase in the risk of developing PNALD. The risk of sepsis is largely attributed to the risk of catheter-related bloodstream infection and bacterial translocation resulting from enteral bacterial overgrowth and underlying intestinal barrier damage. First and foremost, the administration of PN requires an intravenous line to be in place. This line, along with conditions associated with PN, increases the risk of recurrent sepsis. Moreover, in this group of patients, there is mounting evidence to suggest that bacterial translocation from the gut may also be an important source of pathogens. O'Brien et al. showed that translocation of Gram-negative bacteria to the mesenteric lymph nodes and liver was more frequent after massive small bowel resection in mice.

Sepsis has been strongly associated with the development of cholestasis in the setting of PN. Evidence supports the proposal that these effects are mediated through endotoxin and other pro-inflammatory molecules. Sepsis likely causes a systemic inflammation in the liver because of the release of pro-inflammatory cytokines that are activated by endotoxins. Pro-inflammatory cytokines such as TNF-α and IL-1β have been shown to down-regulate the transcription of crucial bile acid transporters. In addition, bacterial lipopolysaccharide acts directly through toll-like receptor 4 to induce pro-inflammatory chemokines and adhesion molecules in activated human hepatic stellate cells, promoting on-going inflammation and fibrosis.

2.4. Bacterial Overgrowth

Many patients receiving PN are at risk of developing small intestinal bacterial overgrowth which may contribute to the development of liver disease. Bacterial overgrowth occurs when large amounts of bacteria normally confined to the colon and lower small bowel populate the upper small intestine.

The reduced enterohepatic circulation that resulted from short bowel syndrome (SBS) and the intestinal stasis that occurs from motility disorders such as chronic intestinal pseudoobstruction predispose many patients receiving PN to small intestinal bacterial overgrowth. It has been postulated that anaerobic bacteria in the small intestine may produce hepatotoxins, such as lithocholic acid, which can lead to hepatic injury. In addition, bacterial overgrowth may contribute to cholestasis by promoting deconjugation of bile acids, which prevents their reabsorption.

2.5. Short Bowel Syndrome

Massive intestinal resection has been identified as a risk factor of PNALD. In one study that used multivariate analysis showed that a small bowel remnant 50 cm in length was significantly associated with chronic cholestasis. Another study of adult long-term PN patients reported that those with the shortest residual intestine were at the greatest risk to develop eventual liver failure and death. Similar results have been shown in pediatric patients with SBS, with up to 70% developing cholestasis. Because SBS causes interruption of enterohepatic circulation and alterations in bile acid metabolism and excretion, it is considered a potential contributing factor in the development of PNALD. Unfortunately, patients with massive small bowel resection are dependent on long-term PN and options are therefore limited when liver failure develops.

2.6. Lack of Enteral Stimulation

PNALD appears more likely to develop in patients who are unable to tolerate any EN compared with those who can tolerate even small amounts. Lack of enteral stimulation had several metabolic and endocrine consequences for intestinal and liver function. One mechanism may be the reduction of food-stimulated release of gastrointestinal hormones such as cholecystokinin (CCK). Biliary sludge can develop due to the reduction of gallbladder contractility and impaired bile flow. A fasting state may also reduce the size of the bile salt pool and bile formation, which can further contribute to the problem. The lower levels of these hormones may also lead to intestinal stasis and consequent bacterial overgrowth another risk factor in PNALD.

2.7. Cyclic Infusion

Cyclic infusion of PN refers to the infusion of a daily supply of PN components over a < 24-hour period (generally 8-12 hours), allowing a period of time off PN. A continuous infusion of PN can result in hyperinsulinemia and fat deposition in the liver, and thereby potentially increase risk of liver complications. Cyclic infusion of PN has been shown to result in a reduction of serum liver enzyme concentrations and conjugated bilirubin concentrations in adult and pediatric patients when compared with continuous infusion. Allowing a period of time each day off PN may reduce the risk of liver complications, especially in patients requiring long-term use.

3. Monitoring

Careful monitoring of patients for identification of PNALD is warranted and should include an evaluation of the biochemical parameters as outlined in Table 2. Frequency of monitoring is generally at least once per week in the adult and pediatric hospitalized patient receiving PN and monthly in the long-term PN patient. In the patient receiving short-term PN therapy, minor increases in serum concentrations of aminotransferases (less than twice the upper limit of the normal reference range) without an elevation of bilirubin are relatively common and generally require no intervention. In this situation, it is sufficient to reevaluate caloric intake to minimize the possibility of overfeeding and follow up with weekly laboratory monitoring. If there is an increase in serum levels of bilirubin or a progressive increase in aminotransferases, alkaline phosphatase, or GGT, then further evaluation is warranted to exclude reversible causes. Because no single laboratory or even histologic finding is definitive for identification of PNALD, it should be based on clinical presentation and exclusion of other diseases.

Elevated serum conjugated bilirubin and GGT concentrations are considered the most sensitive indicators of cholestasis. However, GGT is an enzyme with activity in the kidneys and pancreas, as well as liver, and therefore lacks specificity to liver disease. The same limitation applies to alkaline phosphatase, which is a sensitive marker for biliary obstruction but is also active in bone and will therefore also be increased during bone formation in children. Serum bile acid concentrations have also been proposed as a marker of cholestasis in infants. However, bile acid concentrations have been demonstrated to have no diagnostic advantage to conjugated bilirubin in at least one study done in neonates. Also, because bile synthesis and transport are variable in the infant, a serum bile acid reference range is difficult to establish. Its routine use as a marker for cholestasis is therefore not recommended at this time. The primary marker for cholestasis is conjugated bilirubin because elevated levels reflect a reduction in bile flow. A conjugated bilirubin >2 mg/dL is generally considered a significant indicator of cholestasis. Progressive and sustained elevations of conjugated bilirubin concentrations have been used to predict severity and mortality in patients with PNALD.

Table 2. Suggested laboratory monitoring parameters for PNALD

Parameter	Comment
Aspartate aminotransferase (AST)	Insensitive and nonspecific marker of hepatocellular injury
Alanine aminotransferase (ALT)	Insensitive and nonspecific marker of hepatocellular injury
γ-Glutamyl transpeptidase (GGT)	Sensitive marker of cholestasis, but nonspecific
Alkaline phosphatase	Sensitive marker of cholestasis, but nonspecific
Bilirubin	
Conjugated (direct)	Considered the primary marker of cholestasis (generally defined as 2 mg/dL)
Unconjugated (indirect)	Isolated elevation rarely due to liver disease;
Total	Primarily associated with hemolytic disorders includes both conjugated and unconjugated fractions; both fractions may be elevated in liver disease
Bile acids	Proposed marker of cholestasis, but not routinely used in practice

Liver enzyme elevations have been shown to be of limited predictive value because enzyme release can be blunted when there is little liver parenchyma left to damage. Bilirubin monitoring can serve as a useful indicator to guide when referral to an intestinal transplant center may be warranted. It has been suggested that a total serum bilirubin >3 mg/dL for >3 months despite some enteral nutrition should indicate a need to refer the patient to a transplant center. Latestage indicators of reduced hepatic function include hypoalbuminemia, coagulopathy, and hypoglycemia occurring during PN cycling.

4. Prevention

Prevention of PNALD is difficult, because causation remains somewhat conjectural and risk factors probably assume differing degrees of importance in individual patients.

4.1. Drug Induced Hepatotoxicity Withdrawal

Drug-induced hepatotoxicity is a potential complication of nearly every medication, because the liver is responsible for their metabolism. Injury to hepatocytes may occur either directly or indirectly due to various reactions. Acetaminophen is an example of an agent that causes a direct toxic reaction to the liver and is the leading cause of drug-induced acute liver failure. It accounts for nearly 50% of cases reported from the US Acute Liver Failure Study Group and is the most common drug or toxin leading to liver transplantation for acute hepatic failure. Another drug-induced mechanism for liver damage is alteration of bile flow. Table 3 provides a list of medications that can contribute to cholestatic injury by affecting bile formation or flow. Patients who develop cholestasis while receiving PN should eliminate medications on this list if at all possible.

Besides, herbal medicines are also popular in many countries and are used for a wide variety of clinical conditions, including common colds, anxiety, diabetes, asthma, constipation, allergic rhinitis, Crohn's disease and ulcerative colitis, bronchitis or cough, cardiovascular diseases, depression, dyspepsia, hyperlipidaemia, inflammatory skin conditions, insomnia, irritable bowel syndrome, liver disease, lower urinary tract infections or benign prostatic hyperplasia, menopausal symptoms, obesity, pain, pregnancy, prevention or treatment of cancer, rheumatic conditions and viral infections. In China, herbal medicine consumption had more than 20% of different kinds of drug.

Table 3. List of drugs associated with cholestatic injury

Antimicrobials	Amoxicillin-clavulanate
	Cephalosporins
	Erythromycin and other macrolides
	Nafcillin
	Nitrofurantoin
	Quinolones
	Rifampin
	Tetracycline
	Trimethoprim-sulfamethoxazole
Estrogens and anabolic steroids	Estradio
	amoxifen
	Danazol
Psychotropic agents	Chlorpromazine
	Haloperidol
	Prochlorperazine
	Carbamazepine
	Phenytoin
	Tricyclic antidepressants
	Sertraline
	Fluoxetine
Nonsteroidal antiinflammatory agents	Sulindac
	Diclofenac
	Ibuprofen
	COX-2 inhibitors
Immunosuppressive agents	Cyclosporine
	Azathioprine
	6-Mercaptopurine
Miscellaneous	Terbinafine
	H2-receptor antagonists
	Sulfonylureas
	Rosiglitazone
	Pioglitazone
	Terfenadine
	Antiretroviral therapy to treat HIV
	Warfarin
	Captopril
	Mesalamine
	Infliximab
	Gold compounds

Table 4. List of hepatotoxic herbs and supplements

DHEA/androstenedione	Inositol nicotinate
Boldo	Kava
Chaparral	Pennyroyal oil
Coenzyme Q-10	Red Yeast
Comfrey	Scullcap
Germander	Valerian root

We find most patients with PNALD had the history of herbal medicine, so it is important to identify and eliminate any herbal supplements that may cause hepatotoxicity (listed in Table 4). Because some herbal supplements do not require a prescription and are assumed by many to be nontoxic, their use is often not revealed by the patient and requires specific probing by the clinician.

4.2. Control of Sepsis

Sepsis is a common complication in patients receiving PN, primarily related to the central venous access device. Infection should be aggressively treated and measures should be taken to minimize recurrence. Strict catheter care procedures should be followed in both the hospital and home setting, including minimizing manipulation of the catheter, using proper hand hygiene and aseptic technique when accessing the catheter, using proper site care, and ensuring proper education of catheter care to the patient or caregiver.

Although removal and replacement of a long-term tunneled or implanted central venous access device should be avoided whenever possible, it is also important to recognize those situations when removal is necessary for successful treatment of infection. Efforts to prevent recurrent catheter-related bloodstream infections rely on identifying those situations when successful treatment with antibiotic or antifungal therapy alone is limited.

4.3. Treatment of Bacterial Overgrowth

Treatment of bacterial overgrowth appears to play an important role in preventing and managing PNALD. The enteral administration of antibiotic therapy appears to be more effective than the intravenous route because the intestine is the targeted site for activity. Because anaerobic bacteria normally found in the colon are primarily associated with overgrowth in the intestine, antibiotic agents that target these organisms have been used and include metronidazole, oral gentamicin, oral neomycin, ciprofloxacin, doxycycline, and others. Although the choice of antibiotic is empiric, metronidazole is generally considered the agent of first choice due to its anaerobic coverage. In addition to improvement of liver enzyme and bilirubin concentrations, clinical response may be dramatic from the patient perspective due to resolution of the uncomfortable and embarrassing symptoms noted above. For patients do not respond to a course of metronidazole, switching to another antibiotic may be beneficial. Measures that may be helpful in preventing recurrence of small bowel bacterial overgrowth include avoidance of simple sugars in the diet, avoidance of gastric acid–suppressing agents, and use of probiotic therapy. In addition, for patients with intestinal stasis due to chronic intestinal pseudoobstruction, agents used to enhance motility may be useful in minimizing recurrence of small bowel bacterial overgrowth. Due to octreotide's ability to also inhibit gastric emptying, combination therapy with erythromycin may be beneficial in mitigating this effect.

4.4. Addition of Choleretic Agents

Ursodeoxycholic acid (UDCA) is a naturally occurring hydrophilic bile acid that is the 7-β-epimer of the primary bile acid chenode oxycholic acid. It can increase the biliary secretion of bile acids and the elimination of toxic substances from hepatocytes, decrease the inflammatory response that ultimately results in fibrosis, stimulate secretion of a bicarbonate-rich fluid from cholangiocytes and augment micelle formation, decreasing the toxicity of bile acids on cell membranes.

In 1987, Poupon and colleagues described the first trial of UDCA in treatment of primary biliary cirrhosis. UDCA improves serum liver biochemistry tests, delays histological progression, and delays the development of complications of portal hypertension for primary biliary cirrhosis. However, the preventation of tauroursodeoxycholic acid (TUDCA, 30 mg/kg/d) and cholecystokinin (CCK, 0.04 μg/kg per dose, i.v., every 12 hours for 14 days) on the development of PNALD in neonates were demonstrated by Heubi and Teitelbaum, respectively. Further RCTs from Arslanoglu et al. and Gokmen et al. demonstrated that UDCA significantly decreased serum GGT activity during PN in for the premature neonates. In case reports and a few small studies, 10 to 15 mg/kg/d of UDCA appears to be safe in preventing of PNALD, however, the high-quality RCTs are rare.

4.5. Modification of PN Formulation

A critical review of the PN formulation should be done whenever liver complications develop. Even if the PN therapy does not initiate the complication, it may contribute to or exacerbate the problem. Over-feeding should be avoided, and a trial of decreasing calories may be warranted when energy requirements are unclear. Providing a balanced energy source by adjusting the carbohydrate-to-fat ratio to give more lipid emulsions may improve serum liver enzymes that are elevated due to steatosis. In the patient receiving long-term PN who develops cholestasis, specifically limiting lipid emulsions dose may be beneficial. Although standard guidelines suggest keeping lipid emulsions < 2.5 g/kg/d in adults and children, there is evidence that a lipid emulsions dose > 1 g/kg/d is associated with development of PNALD. Therefore, at least a short-term trial of stopping PNALD or limiting to < 1 g/kg/d appears reasonable.

Although the role that amino acids play in the development of PNALD in the adult and older child is unclear, it does seem to influence the development of cholestasis in the adults and infants. In addition, avoiding high-protein doses may also be beneficial in minimizing risk of developing PNALD. Finally, infusing PN over a cyclic period rather than a continuous, 24-hour infusion rate may be beneficial in reducing the risk of PNALD. A lipid emulsion containing a physical mixture of soybean oil, MCT, olive oil and fish oil (SMOF) and enriched in vitamin E has shown safety and tolerance in surgical patients and premature neonates. First beneficial effects of SMOF with respect to elevated bilirubin levels were reported in infants and children with PNALD.

Klek et al. had demonstrated SMOF was safe and well tolerated over 4 weeks in adults. Infusion of SMOF is effective in modifying the fatty acid composition of both plasma and cellular lipids, with a desirable reduction in ω-6 /ω-3 PUFAs ratio. Meanwhile, the SMOF is benefit for maintaining in parameters of liver function and preventing cholestasis.

4.6. Early Enteral Intake

Because even small amounts of enteral intake may be beneficial in promoting enterohepatic circulation of bile acids, all measures to optimize the enteral route for feeding should be taken. For example, in the patient with chronic intestinal pseudoobstruction receiving continuous gastric decompression, a trial of jejunal feeding at a slow rate during the night may be beneficial. Medications to enhance motility may be necessary to aid success, and multiple attempts may be required before tolerance is achieved. During periods of acute illness, enteral tolerance may be more difficult to achieve and set-backs can be expected, but attempts should be made to restart enteral feeding as soon as possible once the condition has stabilized. Patients with SBS should be encouraged to maximize oral intake because at least some of their intake will be absorbed. These patients may even require a reduction in PN calories in order to prevent unwanted weight gain, but fluid requirements generally remain high because stool output tends to increase when oral intake increases.

4.7. Prophylactic Cholecystectomy

Prophylactic cholecystectomy should be considered in all patients who received long-term PN. However, the preventive effect of prophylactic cholecystectomy for PNALD is still unclear.

5. Treatment

When a patient receiving PN develops liver complications, it is necessary to review all aspects of care to identify and eliminate or treat other factors that may be contributing. It is also important to review the PN formulation and consider modifications that may improve outcome. Table 5 shows the strategies to consider when a patient receiving PN develops PNALD.

5.1. PN Supplementation

Recently, evidence has suggested that lipid emulsion containing fish oil as a novel strategy may be useful in reversing PNALD. Research on animals has shown that fish oil-derived lipid emulsion prevented hepatic steatosis, when compared to conventional soybean oil-based products.

In 1997, Yeh et al. compared groups of rats receiving PN with either a fish oil-based or an ω-6-rich safflower oil-based lipid emulsion. They showed that fish oil-fed rats had reduced superoxide dismutase and glutathione peroxidase activities levels, suggesting that ω-3 PUFAs may play a role in reducing free radicals that contribute to the suppression of the inflammatory pathway. This is consistent with several other studies showing that fish oil modulates inflammation through the inhibition of TNF-α and by the reduction of cytokines that trigger pro-inflammatory reactions.

Table 5. Strategies to manage PNALD

1. Rule out other causes	Hepatotoxic medications Herbal supplements Biliary obstruction Hepatitis Sepsis
2. Consider modifications to parenteral nutrition	Decrease dextrose Decrease IV lipid emulsion to <1 g/kg/d Provide a balance of dextrose and lipid emulsion Cyclic infusion Specialized amino acid formulation in infants
3. Maximize enteral intake	Specialized amino acid formulation in infants Encourage oral diet Tube feeding, even at slow rate
4. Prevent/treat bacterial overgrowth	Enteral antibiotics, such as Metronidazole Gentamicin Neomycin Doxycycline Ciprofloxacin In chronic intestinal pseudoobstruction patients, consider agents to enhance motility Metoclopramide Erythromycin Tegaserod Octreotide
5. Pharmacotherapy	Aggressive treatment of infection Ursodeoxycholic acid (ursodiol) Treatment of pruritus Cholestyramine Rifampin Phenobarbital
6. Intestinal transplantation	Consider for patients with parenteral nutrition failure

In 2005, Gura et al. first reported that two infants with PNALD had significant improvement of liver function and complete resolution of cholestasis after the use of fish oil-based lipid emulsion. Subsequently, a number of small studies demonstrated the beneficial use of fish oil lipid emulsions in treatment of PNALD in infants. A Boston group was first to describe two infants with SBS and PNALD while on prolonged PN using a soybean-based lipid source (Intralipid) who had marked improvement and reversal of cholestasis within 60 d of changing the lipid source to a purely ω-3 fish oil-based emulsion (Omegaven). The American Pediatric Surgery Association's systematic review has recommended that the therapeutic lipid restriction of the standard soybean-based lipid emulsion for neonates with PNALD and the use of fish oil-based lipid emulsions in children with PNALD because it is safe and effective in reversing these conditions. The association has not recommended the use of temporary soybean lipid infusion with enteral fish oil in PNALD due to relatively weak evidence. There is also similarly weak evidence to recommend SMOF or other hybrid lipids in treatment of PNALD.

In children, PNALD largely presents as cholestasis, steatosis is more common than cholestasis in adults. The fish oil-based lipid emulsions successfully reverse the hepatic cholestasis in children, however, it's unclear whether oil-based lipid emulsions reversed the hepatic steatosis in adults. Pironi et al. in 2010 and Jurewitsch et al. in 2011 reported cases of improvement of liver function tests during the use of a fish oil-based lipid emulsion. In our experience, we performed an open-label study of a fish oil-based lipid emulsions in 15 adults with SBS, who developed cholestasis while receiving soybean oil-based lipid emulsion. Our data demonstrated that 12 of the 15 had their DB normalized within 4 weeks and serial liver biopsy specimens showed progressive histological improvement. In addition to cholestatic reversal, a fish oil-based lipid emulsion is associated with significant improvement in all major lipid panels such as total serum cholesterol, triglyceride and high-density lipoprotein. It should also be noted that more research into the long-term outcomes of this novel therapy for PNALD in adults is required. In 2013, Burns and Gill also described an adult home PN patient where use of a fish oil-based lipid emulsion appeared to reverse PNALD.

However, Soden and colleagues reported that treatment with ω-3 fatty acids might not offer complete reversal of liver fibrosis. ω-3 fatty acids can also exert an antiplatelet action and sometimes potentiate risk for bleeding.

Venecourt-Jackson and Walmsley concluded that well-balanced mixture of ω-3, ω-6, and ω-9 fatty acids might be preferable to ω-3-only preparations in PNALD.

How might ω-3 fatty acids improve liver function in PN patients? ω-3 fatty acids probably manifest anti-inflammatory actions by evoking a biochemical shift from ω-6 fatty acid-derived pro-inflammatory eicosanoids to anti-inflammatory forms. The exact mechanism for this is still unclear, although eicosapentaenoic acid and ocosahexaenoic acid may attenuate hepatocyte apoptosis induced by bile acids. NF-κB modulates tumor necrosis factor-α and other pro-inflammatory cytokines that are thought to be involved in these inflammatory processes and whose action is reduced by ω-3 fatty acids. The degree of PN-induced fatty liver may depend on plasma insulin concentrations and the portal insulin to glucagon molar ratio that may be more favorable with ω-3 fatty acids.

Glutamine is a primary fuel for enterocytes and for gut-associated lymphoid tissue. Addition of glutamine to PN solutions may lead to a significant improvement in intestinal epithelium barrier function, by up-regulating the expression of tight junction proteins and reducing the translocation of bacteria from the gut lumen to the systemic circulation. Wang et al. and Wu et al. reported their experience of parenteral glutamine improving outcomes in very low birth-weight infants and infant rabbits. The serum levels of AST and TB decreased after PN in the glutamine-supplemented group. However, intravenous forms of glutamine are not readily available in some countries, since the benefits of treatment remain controversial and guidelines for their use are needed.

5.2. Transplantation

First of all, isolated small intestinal or combined liver-intestinal transplantation should be used cautiously, because survival on intestinal and liver transplantation is less than that on long-term TPN and the advent of fish oil as an emerging treatment. For patients who have established end-stage PNALD and can't wean off TPN, fish oil may not improve established fibrosis, and certainly cirrhosis, so the only option may be transplantation, this has been demonstrated to normalize liver blood test abnormalities in patients receiving an isolated intestinal transplantation. Over the last decade, there have been significant improvements in surgical techniques, organ allocation, immunosuppression and post-transplant care. With the use of anti-lymphoid preparations and minimal post-transplant immunosuppression, the University of Pittsburgh has recently reported that the 1- and 5-year survival rates of intestine-liver allografts were 92% and 70%, respectively. Of the current 272 survivors, 245 (90%) were completely off PN with full nutritional autonomy. Therefore, though it is still associated with significant morbidity and mortality such as infection and chronic rejection, transplantation remains a promising option for patients with end-stage liver disease.

Conclusion

PNALD is a common and potentially life-threatening problem for patients receiving long-term PN. The use of emulsions, particularly those containing phytosterols, is associated with PNALD. Management strategies for its prevention and treatment include consideration of early enteral feeding, reduction of total calories and amount of ω-6 PUFAs, removal of phytosterols, the use of specialized lipid emulsions such as fish oil emulsions, and isolated small intestinal or combined liver-intestinal transplantation. However, whether fish oil is a useful salvage maneuver in adults requires more study even if it is effective in infants, and whether there is a time-window during which the liver can be salvaged, but after which it can't, needs to be determined. In conclusion, a greater understanding of the pathogenesis of PNALD has led to targeted interventions to prevent and treat the condition. Further study should aim to better understand the mechanisms of PNALD and the long-term outcomes of its therapies.

References

[1] Xu ZW, Li YS. Pathogenesis and treatment of parenteral nutrition-associated liver disease. *Hepatobiliary Pancreat. Dis. Int.* 2012; 11(6): 586-93.

[2] Xu Z, Li Y, Wang J, Wu B, Li J. Effect of omega-3 polyunsaturated fatty acids to reverse biopsy-proven parenteral nutrition-associated liver disease in adults. *Clin. Nutr.* 2012; 31(2):217-23.

[3] Wales PW, Allen N, Worthington P, George D, Compher C; the American Society for Parenteral and Enteral Nutrition, Teitelbaum D. A.S.P.E.N. Clinical Guidelines: Support of Pediatric Patients With

Intestinal Failure at Risk of Parenteral Nutrition-Associated Liver Disease. *JPEN J. Parenter. Enteral. Nutr.* 2014 Apr 2.

[4] Nandivada P, Chang MI, Potemkin AK, Carlson SJ, Cowan E, O'loughlin AA, Mitchell PD, Gura KM, Puder M. The Natural History of Cirrhosis From Parenteral Nutrition-Associated Liver Disease After Resolution of Cholestasis With Parenteral Fish Oil Therapy. *Ann. Surg.* 2013 Dec 26.

[5] Lauriti G, Zani A, Aufieri R, Cananzi M, Chiesa PL, Eaton S, Pierro A. Incidence, prevention, and treatment of parenteral nutrition-associated cholestasis and intestinal failure-associated liver disease in infants and children: a systematic review. *JPEN J. Parenter. Enteral. Nutr.* 2014; 38(1):70-85.

[6] Carter BA, Shulman RJ. Mechanisms of disease: update on the molecular etiology and fundamentals of parenteral nutrition associated cholestasis. *Nat. Clin. Pract. Gastroenterol. Hepatol.* 2007; 4(5):277-87.

[7] Rangel SJ, Calkins CM, Cowles RA, Barnhart DC, Huang EY, Abdullah F, Arca MJ, Teitelbaum DH, 2011 American Pediatric Surgical Association Outcomes and Clinical Trials Committee. Parenteral nutrition-associated cholestasis: an American Pediatric Surgical Association Outcomes and Clinical Trials Committee systematic review. *J. Pediatr. Surg.* 2012; 47(1):225-40.

[8] Kumpf VJ. Parenteral nutrition-associated liver disease in adult and pediatric patients. *Nutr. Clin. Pract.* 2006; 21(3):279-90.

[9] Arsenault DA, Potemkin AK, Robinson EM, Fallon EM, Ozonoff A, de Meijer VE, Puder M. Surgical intervention in the setting of parenteral nutrition-associated cholestasis may exacerbate liver injury. *J. Pediatr. Surg.* 2011; 46(1):122-7.

[10] Shu ZJ, Zhang LH, Li JS. Prevention of total parenteral nutrition-induced cholestasis by low non-protein energy supply: an animal experiment and clinical study. *Clin. Nutr.* 1994; 13(4):234-42.

[11] Nandivada P, Carlson SJ, Chang MI, Cowan E, Gura KM, Puder M. Treatment of parenteral nutrition-associated liver disease: the role of lipid emulsions. *Adv. Nutr.* 2013; 4(6):711-7.

In: Parenteral Nutrition
Editor: Shana Lelio
ISBN: 978-1-63321-112-4

Chapter 6

Refeeding Syndrome in Children: Risk Assessment, Diagnostics and Management

Jasna Lenicek Krleza[*1], *Zrinjka Misak*[2], *Oleg Jadresin*[2], *Ana Grzunov*[1] *and Jasminka Stepan-Giljevic*[3]
[1]Children's Hospital Zagreb, Dep. of Laboratory Diagnostics, Zagreb, Croatia
[2]Children's Hospital Zagreb,
Dept. of Pediatric, Referral Center of Pediatric Gastroenterology and Nutrition, Zagreb, Croatia
[3]Children's Hospital Zagreb,
Dep. of Pediatric Oncology and Haematology, Zagreb, Croatia

Abstract

Refeeding syndrome is a well-described state of the series of metabolic and biochemical changes that occur during the supplemental feeding of malnourished patients. The shifts in fluids and electrolytes can lead to complications during artificial feeding and if not recognized and untreated can lead to death. Although the physiology and

* Correspondence: Jasna Lenicek Krleza, Children's Hospital Zagreb, Zagreb, Croatia; e-mail: jlenicek@gmail.com.

pathophysiology is well known, the circumstances under which the syndrome appears, clinical manifestations and management of these patients is less clear. To date, there are no published randomized controlled studies for refeeding syndrome in pediatric population. Published studies are generally lower level of evidence (level 3 and 4) that include cohort studies, case reports and expert opinions.

After the brief report of pathophysiology, we described refeeding syndrome cases from our clinical practice. Mainly, occurrence in pediatric patients has been reported in children with cancer. Then follow the patients with primary gastroenterological or neurological disease in the intensive care unit. In this chapter we describe risk assessment by defining the degree of malnutrition and planning of nutrition support. Baseline biochemical tests and laboratory monitoring, using reference change value of the most important analytes, can identify refeeding syndrome before symptoms appear. In this regard, the refeeding syndrome is laboratory diagnoses that provide a signal for treatment that is significantly simplified and includes termination of feeding, correction of electrolytes and continuation of feeding gradually and slowly.

Introduction

Refeeding Syndrome (RFS) is a set of clinical symptoms (heart, lung, liver, kidney, neurological, metabolic and haematological) that occur as a result of fluid and electrolyte shifts in malnourished patients in response to an inappropriately high-calorie diet. This applies to any form of complementary food after several hours of fasting. It includes enteral or parenteral nutrition, as well as uncontrolled and unlimited oral intake. Changes in fluids and electrolytes are caused by hormonal and metabolic changes that can cause severe complications and death. The main biochemical feature of RFS is hypophosphataemia, although the syndrome is complex and may include a disruption in the balance of water and nitrate content, alterations in the metabolism of glucose, fat and protein, thiamine deficiency, hypokalemia and hypomagnesaemia. These deficiencies vary from case to case. They depend on the severity of the health status of the organism (type and duration of primary disease), on the nutritional status or on the severity of the malnutrition of the organism which suffers from the amount of the retained energy, vitamins and minerals "reserve" as an effect. Their deficiency is visible by measuring their concentrations in the blood. In doing so, a deficiency in all minerals is not necessarily pronounced; all combinations are possible with various severity levels for each. Thus, the symptoms that occur as a consequence of this deficiency are unpredictable and can range from asymptomatic cases to the dysfunction of any of the vital organs; inasmuch as they are not treated (with a correction of electrolyte imbalances) they can cause a coma and death [1-5].

Over the last sixty years, since RFS was first clinically described and published, what we in fact call RFS has still not been clearly defined.

A clear international consensus has not been set as to when we can truly say that RFS has developed, whether this is a laboratory diagnosis, or the moment of onset of clinical symptoms. Laboratory diagnosis refers to the moment when while feeding malnourished patients, decreased concentration of one or more major electrolytes (particularly phosphates) can be observed in the serum, without any symptoms or without any clearly expressed symptoms, while the appearance of symptoms in laboratory findings implies disturbance in vital function that are primarily as results of low blood phosphates [6,7].

In a review of the published literature, we can find individual case reports or reports on series of cases, cohort studies and expert opinions. The level of evidence (LOE) of the published studies is 3 and 4. On this basis, in 2006 the National Institute for Health and Clinical Excellence (NICE) claimed that the recognition and timely inclusion of compensatory mechanisms is essential to reduce, if not completely eliminate the morbidity and mortality associated with this phenomenon. Guidelines for the management of RFS in adults have been published. These guidelines define the criteria for at at-risk and high risk patients (Table 1), as well as instructions for the implementation of compensation mechanisms in case of occurrence of electrolyte deficits. However, in medical practice, RFS still occurs frequently [2,4].

Table 1. Criteria for determining patients at high risk of developing refeeding syndrome

Patient has one or more of the following:	Patient has two or more of the following:
• BMI less than 16 kg/m^2	• BMI less than 18.5 kg/m^2
• unintentional weight loss greater than 15% within the last 3–6 months	• unintentional weight loss greater than 10% within the last 3–6 months
• little or no nutritional intake for more than 10 days	• little or no nutritional intake for more than 5 days
• low levels of potassium, phosphate or magnesium prior to feeding.	• a history of alcohol abuse or drugs including insulin, chemotherapy, antacids or diuretics.

Modified from National Institute for Health and Clinical Excellence (NICE) guideline – Nutrition support in adults) [2]

RFS is generally a term associated with marked malnutrition, primarily with anorexia. However, many clinical conditions represent a risk for RFS. There are three basic groups of patients that are at risk of developing RFS: (1) individuals with a low intake of nutrients, (2) individuals with an increased loss of nutrients, and (3) individuals with a reduced absorption. These groups include a wide range of individuals for whom various medical conditions as well as social, economic and psychological statuses that affect all age groups are responsible for malnutrition and risk [6,7].

The Incidence of Refeeding Syndrome

The lack of a clear definition of RFS entails the lack of randomized controlled trials and published data on its frequency. Moreover, as was already mentioned, often mild symptoms frequently remain unrecognized, and low electrolytes are often associated with secondary diseases. For these reasons, the frequency of RFS remains unknown. According to a study by Camp and Allon, in 10197 hospitalized patients, the incidence of severe hypophosphatemia was 0.43% [8]. The published results of studies on patients who were on total parenteral nutrition (TPP) revealed that 30 to 38% of patients who received phosphate had hypophosphataemia, as did 100% of patients who received no phosphates in the parenteral nutrition [9], while the frequency of RFS in oncological patients was observed in more than 25% of patients [10].

The Pathophysiology and Characteristics of RFS

Under normal circumstances, the body uses glucose as a primary source of energy. This requires a continuous intake of carbohydrates. Two to three hours after the intake of carbohydrates, blood glucose becomes available and is retained as glycogen. The amount of glycogen is limited and provides a short-term source of energy to the body in situations where food intake fails. The body thus retains proteins that would not be used for energy purposes. Excessive food intake, that is, excessive energy intake, is stored by the body as fat, which represents the most important energy reserve in the human body [11].

In a short period of fasting (24 hours), glycogenolysis takes place in the liver and in muscles to compensate for glucose. After the glycogen is expended, the gluconeogenesis process begins. Amino acids from muscle protein and fatty acids from fatty tissues provide the organism glucose as an energy source through metabolic reconstruction. With gluconeogenesis pyruvate and lactate may also provide glucose. This initial fasting period are characterized by increased protein degradation [11].

If fasting continues, the body will slow down and reduce its basal metabolism rate by about 20 to 25%. Most organs and tissues in these conditions switch to fatty acids as an energy source. The brain is the organ that primarily uses glucose, and can only partially switch to ketones as an energy source. By switching to fat as an energy source in the body, protein and muscle mass are maintained. The reduction of the proteolysis rate, an increased migration of fatty acids and formation of ketone is characteristic of this period. In addition, at this stage there is also a decrease in intracellular concentrations of minerals (electrolytes) and vitamins. Serum electrolyte concentrations usually remain normal because of intracellular space contraction, decreased renal excretion and withdrawal from storage in the body. Under these conditions, the body slowly begins to consume itself and this is its mode of survival. Bearing these metabolic changes in mind, they are changes that mostly occur in thin or emaciated and malnourished people. However, they can also occur in overweight people who resort to starvation as a means to decrease their body weight [11].

During the supplemental feeding process, the increase in blood glucose leads to increased insulin secretion and decreased glucagon secretion. This hormonal shift results in the stimulation of the synthesis of glycogen, protein and fat. Minerals such as phosphor and magnesium, as well as cofactors such as thiamine, are necessary for these processes. Insulin stimulates the absorption of potassium and glucose into the cell, and magnesium and phosphates enter the cell. This leads to a reduction in serum concentrations of phosphates, potassium and magnesium which are already in deficit in the body. Clinical symptoms of RFS occur as the result of a lack of these minerals and rapid changes in the basal metabolism rate [1,11].

Phosphor is the primary intracellular mineral. It is found in blood in the form of free and protein-binding inorganic phosphate. It is essential for many intracellular processes: it activates enzymes and messengers, stores energy in the form of adenosine triphosphate (ATP), regulates the affinity of haemoglobin for oxygen and thus regulates the supply of oxygen to the tissues, participates in the regulation of acid-base balance, is an integral part of DNA,

RNA and cellular membranes and is responsible for its integrity. The depletion of phosphor in the whole body occurs in the RFS and insulin secretion leads to increased absorption and utilization of phosphate in the cell. This leads to a deficit of intracellular and extracellular phosphor. In these conditions, even slight decrease in serum phosphate levels can lead to a significant dysfunction of cellular processes that affects virtually every physiological system. Hypophosphatemia is a surrogate marker for RFS, but may be present before the feeding of undernourished patients with malnutrition, in diabetes, alcoholism, or in prolonged severe respiratory alkalosis and in vitally risk patients. Moreover, antacids can also be a cause of hypophosphatemia. [12-14]. Potassium, the main intracellular cation, is also deficient in malnutrition, although its serum concentrations may remain normal. Start of anabolic processes leads to the absorption of potassium into the cell stimulated with insulin, which results in severe hypophosphatemia, changes in electrochemical membrane potential, abnormal heart rhythm and heart failure. Hypokaliemia is probably the most common electrolyte deficit in clinical practice. The causes of hypokaliemia, besides in refeeding, are an increased loss of stool (diarrhea), an increased loss of urine, metabolic alkalosis, or secondarily as a result of taking many drugs (diuretics, β-adrenergic agents, high-dose glucocorticoids, insulin) [12,14,15].

Magnesium, predominantly an intracellular cation, is an important cofactor in most enzyme systems, such as in those involved in oxidative phosphorylation and ATP production. It is essential to the structural integrity of DNA, RNA and ribosomes, it affects the membrane potential of cells and its deficiency can lead to changes in neuromuscular excitability and heart disorders. Besides RFS, where we find acute hypomagnesaemia, the cause of reduced magnesium levels may be diarrhea, pancreatitis, malnutrition, alcoholism, metabolic acidosis, or secondarily as a result of therapy (amphotericin B, furosemide, aminoglycosides, cisplatin, cyclosporin). Hypomagnesaemia can cause hypocalcaemia and hypokalemia (K activator, the ATP-ase pump, and impairs the release of parathyroid hormones). It can also be falsely lowered in cases of significant hypoalbuminemia. The correction of potassium deficiency along with magnesium values (the lower reference range or lower) is not possible without correcting the magnesium. [12,14,16]. Hypocalcaemia is a sign of lower total serum calcium levels and is present relatively often in different states (sepsis, pancreatitis, trauma). Serum calcium concentrations return to normal values 5 to 6 days after recovery from an acute illness. The etiology of hypocalcaemia is multi-factorial and not fully understood. However, the interpretation of findings of total serum calcium may be incorrect in situations where there is markedly reduced albumin, which is often found in malnourished patients. Under conditions in which the concentration of serum albumin is low, it is necessary to determine the ionized calcium level [12,17]. Thiamine deficiency is the most common vitamin deficiency that occurs as a re-alimentation complication. Thiamine is an essential cofactor of key enzymes in the metabolism of carbohydrates and synthesis of ATP. Its deficiency leads to Wernicke's encephalopathy (ataxia, ophthalmoplegia, confusion, hypothermia, coma) or Korsakoff's syndrome (amnesia, confabulation) [4,18].

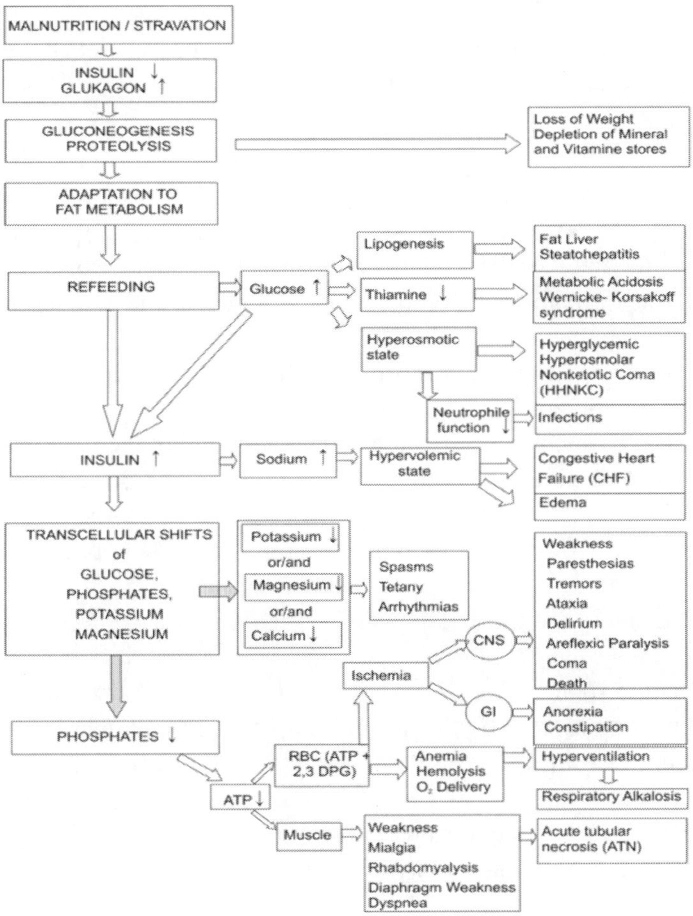

Figure 1. Consequences of the major metabolic and biochemical changes in the refeeding syndrome. Modified from Boateng [1].

Changes in carbohydrate metabolism lead to changes in sodium and water balance. The introduction of carbohydrates in the diet leads to a decrease in the renal excretion of water and sodium. If fluid intake is increased to maintain dieresis, this can lead to fluid overload, congestive heart failure and pulmonary edema [1,3].

An excessive intake of glucose can lead to hyperglycemia, osmotic diuresis and dehydration. There can also be a stimulation of lipogenesis, which can lead to fatty changes in the liver, increased production of carbon dioxide, hypercapnia and respiratory failure [1].

Mutual hormonal and biochemical relations and the consequences that arise during feeding after starvation can be seen in Figure 1 [1].

During fasting, due to the reduced food intake, there is a lack of minerals and vitamins in the body. Nevertheless, through control mechanisms and their redistribution between compartments, concentrations of electrolytes in the blood are mainly normal. Baseline concentrations of electrolytes were measured before refeeding; this is why they are not a true reflection of the state of the organism. Reduced basal electrolyte concentration values can be found when due to other disturbances compensatory mechanisms are no longer sufficient. The principle of complementary foods in such cases requires a specific approach, but is basically clear.

Laboratory monitoring during the supplemental feeding of malnourished patients are an integral part of NICE guidelines and come in the form of protocols. The protocols include biochemical tests along with the dynamics of definition and also note explanations and interpretations. These protocols were developed by Guideline Development Group (GDP), on the basis of good practice point (GPP) and as a recommendation for the best practice based on experience (LOE 3 or 4) and/or formal consensus [2,3]. According to this protocol, laboratory monitoring includes:

1 Sodium, potassium, urea and creatinine for the assessment of renal functions as well as the status of water, sodium and potassium. The interpretation of results includes insight on therapies and fluid balance.
   a) After the initial values, the dynamics of determination include monitoring once a day until the results are stable, and then 1 to 2 times a week.
   b) Sodium and potassium in the urine can be useful and necessary in monitoring and replenishing electrolytes which are lost gastrointestinally.

2 Glucose for monitoring glycaemia and due to possible resistance to glucose, which is not a rare occurrence.
   a) After the initial value, values need to be determined twice a day or more if necessary, until the results are stable; then they are to be determined once a week.

3 Magnesium and phosphates in the body are often depleted despite initial values that are often within the reference range.
   a) After the initial values are determined, once a day during the first week (there is risk of developing RFS), then 2 to 3 times a week until the values are stable, then once a week.

4 Liver function tests including International Normalised Ratio (INR): deviation of normal values is common, although the reasons can be complex and should be interpreted taking this into consideration. Deviation in laboratory tests could be a result of parenteral nutrition, sepsis or other disorders.
   a) The initial values are determined, then twice a week until values are stable, then once a week.

5 Calcium and albumin: a possible presence of hypo and hypercalcemia. Albumins are not a measure of the status of protein, rather a measure of malnutrition or disease. It is necessary to correct serum calcium levels (because of albumin).
   a) The initial values are determined, then once a week.

6 C-reactive protein (CRP) is necessary to assess the presence of acute phase reaction. The CRP value is important in interpreting, but can also be helpful in assessing the results of other parameters (proteins, trace elements, vitamins).
   a) The initial values are determined; then 2 to 3 a week until results are stable.

7 Zinc and copper, trace elements, are often lacking in malnutrition. When interpreting the results it should be borne in mind that the acute phase (an elevated CRP level) can be reflected in a reduced zinc level and an increased copper level.
   a) The initial values are determined, then, depending on the results, again every 2 to 4 weeks.

8 Selenium deficiency is found in severe disease and sepsis, but also in long-term nutrition support. The acute phase lowers selenium values.
   a) Is determined only when a deficiency is suspected, and further determinations depend on the initial one.

9 Complete blood count (CBC) and MCV: Anaemia due to iron or folic acid deficiency is common in malnourished patients. Sepsis significantly affects the results of the CBC.
   a) The initial values are determined; then 1 to 2 times a week until results are stable, then once a week.

10 Iron and ferritin. Iron deficiency is common in long-term parenteral nutrition. When interpreting the results, the acute phase reaction should be paid close attention to, when the iron is reduced and ferritin elevated.
   a) The initial values are determined, then again every 3 to 6 months.

11 Folate, B12: Serum folate/B12 sufficient, with full blood count.
   a) The initial values are determined, then again every 2 to 4 weeks.

12 Manganese and 25-OH vitamin D. These tests are rarely needed, unless there is cause for concern [2,3].

RFS from a Laboratory Perspective

The dynamics of laboratory monitoring of these patients according to the protocols of published guidelines (NICE, 2006) [2] allows the identification of the development RFS before the onset of symptoms and with the correction of deficiency symptoms are prevented from being developed. In this respect, RFS is a laboratory diagnosis. This understanding includes laboratory professionals in and commits them to the team that treats and cares for such patients. What can a laboratory expert do in this regard? What is important for good laboratory monitoring? How can he or she help a physician in interpreting the laboratory test results?

From a laboratory perspective, the most important feature of RFS is the rapid and uncertain change in the concentration of glucose and electrolytes in serum, which depends on the applied therapeutic procedure. These treatments are generally not known to the laboratory professional, and neither is the weight of the underlying disease, which may or may not be present.

Standardized methods of determination, standardized complete pre-analytical procedures and analytical phases of laboratory practice, as well as the implementation of quality control are the basic requirement for good laboratory practices (according to ISO 15189). Laboratory errors were thus reduced to a minimum. The interpretation of the laboratory test results is part of the post-analytical phase, and it is common to both biochemists and clinicians.

In medical practice, most often the obtained laboratory tests results are compared with the reference values (according age and gender of patients). This is the so-called longitudinal evaluation of laboratory test results. It is based on a comparison of the obtained values of the analyte with the previous result. The usefulness of such assessments in laboratory monitoring may be calculated through an index of individuality (II) for each analyte. It represents the ratio of inter-individual (CVi) and intra-individual variability (CVintra). The smaller the ratio (II), the more pronounced the individuality of each analyte is, and hence the usefulness of the reference interval lessens [19,20].

Laboratory monitoring is used to monitor the effects of therapeutic procedures on the health status of patients. This means that the assessment of laboratory test results is relevant to the comparison of the obtained values to the preceding results. The slightest differences between two obtained concentrations in the required medical reports that could be linked to actual changes in the patient's medical status are referred to as critical differences, or reference change values (RCV). RCV or critical difference values represent the minimum change required analyte that will lead to changes in patient status. It involves biological (CV_i) and analytical variation (CVa) The formula and method of calculating the RCV according to Ricos and colleagues can be found in literature [19]. The database containing biological and analytical variations is continually updated and is available on the website [21]. Ricos and colleagues calculated the RCV values for 216 analytes [22], while Table 2 shows the RCV values for laboratory tests that are used in the daily laboratory monitoring of RFS [47]. The RCV values were calculated from changes in healthy subjects, and were present with probability level 95%, provided that the CVa < CVi (approximately CVa/CVi=0.5). RCV values in diseased states in individual analytes were significantly higher, although studies have shown that RCV in diseased and healthy states do not significantly change [20,22,23]. However, in clinical terms, this is not significant because it is better to register the change, and then to decide that this is clinically unimportant, rather than to ignore the change in the patient's condition. Furthermore, the analytical imprecision of the CVa is replaced by the desired analytical quality specifications that is based on CVi 0.5. Of course, a prerequisite for this is the daily implementation of internal quality control on the laboratory's analytical phase to achieve the desirable specifications for imprecision, inaccuracy and allowable total error [21]. For the proper interpretation of the laboratory test results, knowledge of the possible interferences is also necessary. It is particularly important to reduce the impact of all the factors from the preanalytical phase on the results (potential errors in blood tests, transport conditions, separation, sample storage)[20,23]. This is done by introducing clear and precise protocols in and outside of the laboratory, and is based on guidelines published by the Clinical and Laboratory Standards Institute (CLSI) and the World Health Organization (WHO) [24,25]. Furthermore, the effects of the most common interferences (haemolysis, icterus, lipemia) should be clearly defined, as well as other known interferences (drugs), or states in which the analytes can be altered.

Table 2. Biological (intra- and interindividual) variation, analytical variation, index of individuality and reference change values for analytes in daily monitoring of refeeding syndrome [47]

Analyte	CV_i (%)	CV_{intra} (%)	Index of individuality (II) (CV_i/CV_{intra})	CV_a Desirable (%)	$RCV_{95\%}$ Desirable specification ($CV_a \sim 0.5CV_i$)(%)
Phosphate	8.5	9.4	0.90	4.3	26.3
Potassium	4.8	5.6	0.86	2.4	14.9
Magnesium	3.6	6.4	0.56	1.8	11.2
Calcium	1.9	2.8	0.68	1.0	5.9
Calcium ionized	1.7	1.9	0.89	0.9	5.3
Sodium	0.7	1.0	0.7	0.4	2.2
Glucose	4.9	6.1	0.80	2.5	15.2

Legend: CV_i intra-individual coefficient of variation; CV_{intra}: inter-individual coefficient of variation; CV_a: desirable coefficient of analytical variation; $RCV_{95\%}$: reference change values at probability level of 95%.

The determination of the initial or basic values of all laboratory parameters provided by the working diagnosis is of great importance. These are values that are determined prior to any therapeutic or diagnostic procedure.

The longitudinal assessment of the initial laboratory tests allows a series of therapeutic procedures. It also presents a comparative value along with the value of the next scheduled laboratory monitoring point.

Refeeding Syndrome in Children

The term RFS in children is mainly associated with marked malnutrition, primarily with anorexia. However, many clinical conditions represent a risk for RFS. Only a few recent reports describe the occurrence of RFS in children: some expert suggestions for reducing the risk of development of RFS in children and recent reports of RFS occurring in children with celiac and Crohn disease [9,26,27,28].

So, why is it that for well-known pathophysiology of RFS, does not exist enough strong studies providing evidence for the clear guidelines for the management of RFS in children? The reasons is probably lack of clear consensus on 1) the most accurate criterion for defining the nutritional status of children [29] and 2) the definition of RFS [6,30].

Though, year 2009, the Guideline for children was published by Cape Town Metropole Paediatric Interesting Group [31].

In this chapter, we present incidence of RFS in children with malignant brain tumors in our hospital during a period of two years. Also, we present two cases of RFS in severe malnourished children. The etiology of their malnutrition is different: celiac disease and cerebral palsy. Through a detailed presentation of the clinical course and laboratory processing, we wanted to emphasize the importance of proper dynamics, and interpretation of results of laboratory tests. In this way it is possible to avoid development of symptoms by timely identifing development of RFS and with the proper correction of electrolyte imbalance.

Degree of malnutrition was defined according to WHO recommendations [17] by the Z-score classification system. The Z-score system expresses the anthropometric value as a number of Z-scores below the reference median value. It was calculated as: (measured value - average value in the reference population) / standard deviation of the reference population. The database uses the National Center for Health Statistics (NCHS) growth reference, so-called NCHS/WHO international reference population, as a basis for comparison across countries. The WHO Global Database on Child Growth and Malnutrition uses the Z-score cut-off point of <-2 SD to classify as moderate and <-3 SD to define severe undernutrition. For calculation we used software Growth Analyser v.3.5.202, by Dutch Growth Foundation.

Refeeding Syndrome in Children with Malignat Brain Tumors

High-risk brain tumors require intensive oncological treatment (surgery, radiotherapy, mega therapy). Illness and intensive care often lead child into a state of malnutrition. With increased laboratory monitoring, treatment involves intensive supportive therapy.

During two years we monitored 30 children with a diagnosis of high-risk malignant brain tumors. We analyzed changes in body weight and body mass index during the implementation of treatment. Applied supportive nutritional therapy was followed by an intensive laboratory monitoring of glucose and acid-base status (ABS). Furthermore, monitoring of electrolyte (phosphate, potassium, magnesium, and calcium), proteins (total proteins, albumin) and metabolites (urea, creatinine) has been made in terms of possible development of the RFS. At last, during two years, data were compared with the outcome of the disease. In the group of children with depletion of body weight, body mass index and evidence changes in laboratory values (phosphate, potassium, magnesium, calcium) has been registered worse outcome of disease. In patients with small changes in the body weight and the body mass index and appropriate laboratory test results we found better outcome of disease. Results in summary are shown in Table 3 [32].

Table 3. Overview of refeeding syndrome frequencies and electrolytes changes in children with malignant brain tumors (32)

	Frequency n (%)
Stable disease	5 (16,7%)
Complete remission	5 (16,7%)
Partial remission	2 (6,7%)
Death of disease	17 (56,6%)
Progression of disease	1 (3,3%)
Average of age	9,8 y (range 2,1y - 18 y)
Female	11 (36,7%)
Male	19 (63,3%)
Normal serum phosphates	8 (26,7%)
Mild hypophosphatemia*	21 (70%)
Mild hypophosphatemia with other electrolytes imbalance	16/21(76,2%)
Severe hypophosphatemia**	1 (3,3%)
Average of correction time: 9,9 days with the exception of two cases – one with very long time of correction and one with unsuccessful correction	

Legend: * *Mild hypophosphatemia:* concentration of serum phosphates is same or under reference intervale according gender and age

***Severe hypophosphatemia*: concentration of serum phosphates is under 0,3 mmol/L

The WHO Global Database on Child Growth and Malnutrition uses a Z-score cut-off point of <-2 SD to classify low weight-for-age, low height-for-age as moderate and severe undernutrition, and <-3 SD to define severe undernutrition.

Case Reports

Our case reports are published [33], but in this chapter we present it in extension.

Case 1: boy aged 8 years and 10 months, due to worsening of general condition and the suspicion of celiac disease was admitted to the Gastroenterology Department and stayed in hospital three weeks.

Case 2: 10 years old girl with cerebral palsy admitted at the Pediatric Emergency Department, stayed in the hospital two weeks.

Solutions used for rehydration and nutrition in this two cases are shown in the Table 4.

Table 4. Compositions of rehydration and feeding solutions used in two case reports

Solution	Solution composition
A	Total parenteral nutrition (TPN) was composed by two solutions. Solution I: glucose, amino acids, fat, potassium, sodium, calcium, phosphorus, magnesium, water, and Solution II: Lipofundin (B. Braun Melsungen AG, Luxemburg) by adding Vitalipida (Fresenius Kabi AG, Germany) and Soluvita (Fresenius Kabi AG, Germany). Composition of these solutions is prescribed by a nutritionist.
B	Continuous parenteral nutrition (glucose, potassium chloride, sodium chloride, calcium chloride, trace elements (Peditrace, Fresenius Kabi AG, Germany), fat (Intralipid, Fresenius Kabi, Sweden), vitamins (Soluvit, Fresenius Kabi AG, Germany), amino acids (Aminoven, Fresenius Kabi AG, Germany)
C	Enteral Nutrition (oral): Pediasure (Abbott Healthcare Pvt Ltd, India)
D	Enteral Nutrition (gluten and lactose free for oral and nasogastric tube feeding): Peptamen (Nestlé HealthCare Nutrition, Switzerland) diluted with water in ratio 1:1 or 1:2).
E	Intravenous rehydration solution (glucose, potassium and calcium chloride, sodium bicarbonate).
F	Intravenous solution for the correction of phosphate: glucose and sodium glycerophosphate pentahydrate (Glycophos, Fresenius Kabi AG, Germany).

Clinical Course and Laboratory Test Results

Case 1

At hospital admission the boy was undernourished, listless and pale with psoriatic skin changes on the limbs. Six months before, he had lost weight and had often diarrhea and vomiting. His body mass (BM) was 17.1 kg (Z score: -4.3), body height (BH) 125.5 cm (height Z score: -1.2) and body mass index

(BMI) 10.9 kg/m^2 (Z score -6.8). Results of the basic laboratory tests showed a marked metabolic acidosis, severe hypokalemia and hypocalcemia and the boy was admitted to the ICU. On the first day, with intravenous rehydration process (solution E), oral feeding was started (solution C, ratio 1:1). On the second day, central venous catheter and nasogastric tube were set and the continuous parenteral (Solution B) and enteral nutrition on the nasogastric tube were introduced (solution D, because IgA anti-tissue transglutaminase antibodies test, AT-tTG, was positive). Metabolic acidosis, K and Ca deficits was corrected gradually through the five days with a daily monitoring of ABS, K and ionized Ca.

Table 5. Laboratory tests results in boy with celiac disease (Case 1) [33]

		1st day*	2nd day	3rd day	4th day	5th day**	6th day	7th day	8th day	10th day	13rd day	19th day
	Hospital department	gastro /IUC	ICU	ICU	ICU	ICU/ gastro	gastro	gastro	gastro	gastro	gastro	gastro
Analyte (units)	Reference range											
Glucose (mmol/L)	3.9 - 5-9	4.0	N	N	N	N	N	N	N	N	N	4.5
Potassium (mmol/L)	3.6 - 5.0	**2.1**	**2.9**	**3.1**	N	N	N	N	N	N	N	4.1
Sodium (mmol/L)	135 - 144	137	N	N	N	N	N	N	N	N	N	139
Phosphate (mmol/L)	1.11 – 1.73	**1.07**				**0.28**	**0.49**	**0.50**	**0.74**	**0.97**	N	1.72
Calcium (mmol/L)	2.16 – 2.63	**1.82**				**1.96**	**1.97**	**1.93**	**2.04**	**2.14**	N	2.26
Ionized calcium (mmol/L)	1.22 – 1.37	**1.16** **1.12**	**1.11**	N								
Magnesium (mmol/L)	0.74 – 0.97	0.70				N	**0.72**	N	N	N	N	0.77
Albumine (g/L)	42 - 51	**28.8**				**26**						
pH (pH units)	7.35 - 7.45	**7.14/** 7.34	N	N	N	N	**7.50**	**7.51**	**7.49**	**7.47**	N	
Hydrogen carbonate (mmol/L)	22 -26	12.5/ 15.5	N	N	N	N	**28.0**	**31.6**	**29.3**	**30.0**	**26.5**	
Base excess(BE)(mmol/L)	-4 do 2	**-16.2/ -11.7**	**-7.9/ -7.1**	N	N	**3.6**	**4.0**	**7.8**	**5.4**	**6.2**	N	
Urea (mmol/L)	2.7 – 6.8	**1.0**										
Creatinine (µmol/L)	46 - 80	**33**										
CRP (mg/L)	0.1 – 2.8	**37.0**			**3.0**	N				N	N	0.2

Legend: N normal value of laboratory test results; Bold: value of laboratory test results (without reference intervals)

* 1st day: Due to the presence of high metabolic acidosis boy is moved to the ICU, introduced intravenous rehydration.

** 5th day: Severe hypophosphataemia reflection of refeeding syndrome.

On the third day of parenteral nutrition the body temperature and blood pressure was dropped. Because bradycardia was observed, and electrocardiogram (ECG) was done (ECG: low T waves, tremor of isoelectric line). Electroencephalogram (EEG) was irregular, too. The laboratory tests were requested and results of them showed a severe hypophosphatemia and hypocalcemia. Gradually, through the three days, phosphates were corrected (solution F). Corrections of electrolytes deficites was monitored daily. On fourth day, TPN (solution A) and gluten free enteral nutrition (solution D) during the day and night (nasogastric tube with enteral pumps) were introduced. Laboratory monitoring (Gluc, ABS, K, Na, Cl, Ca, P, Mg) through the first week of TPN and enteral feeding was done every day. Next week, same laboratory tests were done twice. Until discharge from hospital, results of laboratory tests were within the reference interval. During the second week of stay, gastroscopy and duodenal biopsy was preformed. Histopathological findings confirmed celiac disease (total villous atrophy on duodenal biopsy and destructive lesion, hypertrophic cysts and increased number of intraepithelial lymphocytes).

Results of laboratory tests were clearly diagnosis of RFS after five day from the start of feeding, after start gluten-free diet: severe hypophosphatemia, hypocalcaemia (partially corrected) and still a low concentration of serum albumin, urea and creatinine. The workflow of laboratory tests results are shown in Table 5. Before leaving the hospital, the boy was 21.3 kg.

Case 2

At the hospital admission, a girl with cerebral palsy was pale, grossly emaciated and undernourished. Her BM was 11.2 kg (below 10th percentile for children with cerebral palsy, weight Z score for general population -7.9), BH 109 cm (height Z-score -3.4), BMI 9.4 kg/m^2 (BMI Z score -9.5). Initial laboratory tests included CBC, and first test results showed a very low concentration of hemoglobin (27 g/L). She received transfusion of two packs of red blood cells in ICU. In view of poor oral intake and diarrhoea that she had from the one day of the admission, she was given partial parenteral nutrition together with enteral nutrition by nasogastric tube. In this case, first venous blood sample was taken for biochemical parameters when parenteral and enteral nutrition already begun (solutions B and C) and red blood cell transfusions was ended. During the first day of feeding, her serum concentrations of P, Mg and K dropped to reflect RFS. Calcium concentration was on the low limit of reference interval. Supplements of phosphoruos, potassium and magnesium were started and the electrolyte concentrations normalised gradually. Also, oral iron therapy was introduced by haematologist. Laboratory monitoring during the first week of parenteral and enteral nutrition included daily determination of K, Na, Cl, Ca, P, Mg in the sample of venous blood, and haematologic parameters (CBC) in sample from capillary blood. After five days of successful correction of electrolyte imbalance and stabilized values of haematological parameters, enteral nutrition was progresivelly increased while parenteral nutrition decreased and finally stopped. The girl started to gain weight. During the second week, laboratory monitoring was performed every second day. After the fourth day, since the clinical status of the girl was stabile, control of laboratory tests (CBC, ABS, K, Na, Ca ionized) was made from capillary blood samples.

In our Case 2, RFS started to develop after the first day of introduced parenteral nutrition. There was a laboratory diagnosis of RFS as mild hypophosphatemia with decreased concentration of the other electrolytes: K, Mg, Ca. At this early stage, symptoms were not expressed, and the correction is obtained on the next three day with the exception of the total Ca concentration, which reached normal levels after two days, and ionized Ca after four days.

Hematological parameters of red blood cells remained stable but although still low. At release from hospital, the girl had 13.5 kg. The workflow of laboratory tests results are shown in Table 6. Parents were instructed about the future girl's nutrition from the nutritionists. Two months after hospitalization, the girl has gained in weight 2.3 kg.

Except severe malnutrition in both cases, these cases showed a critical condition for which their treatment begins in the ICU, where children with brain tumors had variability condition and BMI depends on stage of disease and treatment. Treatment and feeding of our two patients in the ICU triggered RFS and the biochemical hallmark feature was hypophosphataemia. According to published literature, 20-40% of adult patients in the ICU has expressed hypophospatemia [34,35]. In pediatric population, published studies show that the frequency of hypophosphatemia, have significantly higher incidence (61%), of which 15% of children developed hypophosphatemia during their stay in the ICU. Statistically significant association with the present hypophosphatemia was malnutrition ($p=0.02$, $OR=3.96$, $CI=1.19-13.3$)

[36]. Other biochemical parameters that reflected RFS also show high incidence in the pediatric ICU: 47.4% for hypomagnesemia, 24.5% for hypocalcemia and 51.9% for hyperglycemia [37]. Yet, despite all precautions when introducing parenteral nutrition in malnourished patients and knowledge about the risk of developing RFS, phosphates often remain „forgotten“ [4]. So, in our two cases, laboratory monitoring during treatment in the ICU also "forgot" in first place phosphates, same as magnesium and RFS in our two cases was not noticed until after the transfer of patients to Department of Gastroenterology where were performed extensive laboratory tests. In Case 1 it was the fifth day, and in Case 2 after the first day from the started parenteral and enteral nutrition. The concentration of serum phosphate on the fifth day was 0.79 mmol / L (73.8%) lower than the initial value in Case 1. In Case 2, we haven't initial value because the sample of venous blood on admission was not acceptable for the required tests (distinct hemolysis and a very small volume of blood). A new sample of venous blood was taken the next day, when parenteral nutrition has begun and when RBC transfusion was completed. Serum phosphate concentration was lower for 0.43 mmol/L (38.7%) than the lower limit of the reference interval.

Table 6. Laboratory test results in girl with cerebral palsy (Case 2)(33)

		1st and 2nd day*	3rd day**	4th day	5th day	6th day	7th day	9th day	14th day	two months later
	Hospital department	ICU	gastro	gastro	gastro	gastro	gastro	gastro	gastro	up visit
Analyte (units)	Reference range	Before /after red cell concentrates	Start feeding						BW 13,5 kg	BW 15 kg
Glucose (mmol/L)	3.9 - 5-9		**6.1**				N	N	N	
Potassium (mmol/L)	3.6 - 5.0		**2.7**	**3.0**	N	N	N	N	N	
Sodium (mmol/L)	135 - 144		139	N	N	N	N	N	N	
Phosphate (mmol/L)	1.11 – 1.73		**0.68**	**0.71**	**0.80**	N	N		N	
Calcium (mmol/L)	2.16 – 2.63		**2.09**	**2.15**	N	N	N	N	N	

Table 6. (Continued)

Ionized calcium (mmol/L)	1.22 – 1.37		**1.13**	**1.17**	**1.19**	**1.21**	N	N	N	
Magnesium (mmol/L)	0.74 – 0.97		**0,71**	N	N	N	N		N	
Albumine (g/L)	42 - 51		**30**				**31**		**32**	
Red Blood Cells (RBC) ($x10^{12}$/L)	4,3 - 5,5	2.2/2.4 3.5/3.8	**3.8**		**4.0**		**3.8**		N	4.9
Haemoglobin (g/L)	121 - 145	27/28 74/82	**81**		**85**		**80**		**105**	124
MCV (fL)	76,5 92,1	51/51 -69/69	**68**		**70**		**72**		N	79
MCH (pg)	24,3 31,5	12/12 -21/22	**21.4**		**21.2**		**21.1**		**24**	25
MCHC (g/L)	304 - 346	239/231 312/318	315		**300**		**295**		N	336
Platelets ($x10^9$/L)	150 - 450	659/601 555/507	**501**		**500**		**477**		429	323
White blood cells (WBC) ($x10^9$/L)	5 - 13	22/23 24/23	**15.9**		**15.3**		N		N	8.8
CRP (mg/L)	0.1 – 2.8		**14.1**				**5.0**		0.5	
pH (pH units)	7.35 - 7.45		**7.495**	N	N	N	N	N	N	
Hydrogen-carbonate (mmol/L)	22 -26		25	N	N	N	N	N	N	
Base excess (BE)(mmol/L)	-4 do 2		0.6	N	N	N	N	N	N	
Urea (mmol/L)	2.7 – 6.8		**1.6**				N		N	
Creatinine (μmol/L)	46 - 80		**33**				**31**		**30**	

Legend: N normal value of laboratory test results; Bold: value of laboratory test results (without reference intervals)

* 1st day: severe anemia and suspected haematemesis treated with transfusion of red cell concentrates (two packs). In Table present hematology parameters before and after transfusion.

** 3rd day: hypophosphataemia, hypokaliemia, hypomagnesiemia - a reflection of refeeding syndrome

Degree and classification of electrolyte deficits in children is not clearly established. According to the published studies, diagnosis of hypophosphatinemia and other serum electrolytes used lower limits of reference range for the cut-off points. Researches on the degree of hypophosphatemia have shown that children older than 5 years have the same classification as adults. In adults, hypophosphatemia is classified as mild (0.64-0.8 mmol/L), moderate (0.32-0.64 mmol/L), and severe (<0.32 mmol/L) [23-25]. According to this classification, hypophosphatemia in Case 1 is marked as "severe hypophosphatemia," and in Case 2 as a "mild hypophosphatemia".

Evaluation of Laboratory Tests

Longitudinal evaluation of results is useful for monitoring of efficiency in therapy since the development of RFS is based solely on laboratory monitoring In Case 1, the initial values of phosphates were on low limit of the reference interval for age. On the fifth day of parenteral nutrition was determined by laboratory diagnosis of severe hypophosphatemia. At this point, the fall in serum phosphate concentration was 73.8% of the initial value, and this is significantly higher than RCV for phosphate. With a probability of 95% we can assess that change has occurred in patient status. The clinical symptoms (hypothermia, changes in ECG and EEG) have appeared the third and fourth days of the admission and start feeding (1-2 days after starting a gluten-free diet), and were attributed to celiac crisis. We assess that these symptoms are reflection of the RFS and that are developed on the second or third day of introduction of gluten free diet. In this moment, difference in phosphate concentration of the initial value, probably was greater than its RCV (> 26.3%). All analytes have a difference between the initial value and the value of the fifth day (difference,%), greater than RCV, but the correction K, Gluc, Ca and ABS was carefully monitored and adjusted daily. Their differences in concentrations from day to day were less or equal to RCV with the exception of glucose on second and third days. Although glucose is within the reference interval, the difference is greater than the RCV. That day was introduced gluten free diet, and glucose starts to rise and shift phosphate into cells. Corrected ABS (pH and concentration of hydrogen carbonate) contribute to decrease in serum phosphate concentration and symptoms appeared on the fourth day (Table 5.). However, the case report of girls with Crohn's disease [9], describes the sudden drop in phosphate on fifth day since the beginning of feeding (63.5% of the previous day) regardless of the daily phosphate supplementation. Changes of phosphate (RCV, our calculations) amounted to 14.3% (second day) and 25% (fourth day). Although the second day phosphate concentrations fell below the lower limit of the reference interval, the diagnosis of RFS was not made until the fifth day (RCV> 26.3%). Furthermore, the description of the case in abandoned child, phosphate decreased for 65.7% in the period of just 12 hours after the start of nutrition and supplementation of phosphate [38]. Recent literature data of the other two cases described RFS in children with Crohn's disease [26], as well as other cases of children with celiac diseases [9], referred concentrations of phosphate (and other analyte) only in a time when values are below the lower limit of the reference interval and do not present comparative values of serum phosphate and other characteristic electrolytes for development of RFS.

How important is proper evaluation of child's status is evident from our first case. RFS and celiac crisis are not completely defined, the symptoms can be very similar but the treatment is very different. RFS treatment involves gradual correction of electrolyte imbalance with reduced food intake compared with celiac crisis, which is treated with corticosteroids. In addition to this, we should keep in mind that coticosteroid therapy may contribute to the further development of already existing RFS (corticosteroids stimulate gluconeogenesis and consequently increase glucose in blood), which can have fatal consequences [27].

A low concentration of albumin in serum isn't indicators of RFS. Although the first 24 hours of fasting, when albumin synthesis a significant decrease, it isn't reflected in serum concentrations because albumin shift from extravascular in the intravascular department. Furthermore, prolonged fasting, due to the contraction of volume, protein concentration in the blood may be higher. Low concentrations of serum albumin are a measure of chronic malnutrition. This is result of gastrointestinal diseases and kidney diseases, which leads to loss of albumin through the intestines or kidneys. Furthermore, inflammatory disease decrease serum albumin due to increased degradation decreased synthesis and increased permeability of capillaries. In this way, extravascular albumin crosses departments. Once albumin was synthesized and release into the circulation, he has a half-time approximately 20 days. That is the reason why albumins are not good indicators of nutritional status. [39]. Our results in both cases confirmed this. During treatment and feeding, the concentration of albumin was not significantly changed. Determination of albumin concentration before feeding has a purpose as the initial value for comparison with the results an extended period as an indicator of malnutrition.

Better indicators of nutritional status are the proteins with shorter half-life. The pre- albumin, whose half-life is 2 days, is very sensitive and specific to changes in the nutritional status. Changes in the pre-albumin concentration can be seen already during the first week of feeding [9,40].

Urea is the end product of protein metabolism, whereas creatinine reflects muscular mass. In severe malnourished patients both parameters were lower, like in our two cases and published cases [9,27].

CRP - inflammatory parameter was slightly elevated in case 1, which is a reflection of celiac disease, and decreased to normal values on the third day of introduction of gluten-free diet. The literature describes cases of transient hypophosphatemia in acute inflammatory diseases with high CRP levels [36,41].

Blood samples for serological tests in celiac disease were taken in the first days of receipt. During the first week, At-tTG was positive (21.7 AU; positive >7 AU), and total serum immunoglobulin A (IgA) was elevated (3.35 g/L, reference interval: 0.4-2.4 g/L). The results of anti-gliadin antibodies (AGA) (IgG, IgA classes) and antiendomysial antibodies tests (EMA) (IgA class) were also positive: index for IgA AGA = 33.7 (positive: >20), for AGA IgG index = 58.3 (positive: >15) and EMA = 2+ (positive). In January this year, the new diagnostic criteria for the diagnosis of celiac disease have been published proposing that celiac disease does not necessarily have to be confirmed by biopsy [42]. In our case, diagnosis of celiac disease was set on the basis of deep duodenal mucosal biopsies according to diagnostic criteria that were applicable at that time (2008) and by whom the diagnosis of celiac disease could be established only by biopsy [43]. In addition, published results in children with celiac disease show strongly positive titer of At-tTG (> 100 AU) [44-46]. Our result, in comparison with these results, is slightly positive. Furthermore, results of AGA and EMA were completed after biopsy was preformed and diagnosis of celiac disease was confirmed. The published results that described a series of 5 cases in children with celiac disease and RFS, cited two cases with the At-tTG > 300 and three cases with positive EMA. The same article does not specify the method and the unit, and in all cases were performed biopsy [27].

Instead of a conclusion of our two cases presented, we agree with the fact that the RFS is initially usually asymptomatic and may go unrecognized [6,26]. Therefore, in this initial phase, laboratory diagnosis is the only indicator of development of RFS. Treatment and nutrition of undernourished patients should not start before the initial concentration of Gluc, K, Na, P, Mg, Ca, Cl, ABS, CBC are done. The same laboratory parameters should be monitored daily during the first week of nutrition, and during the second week every 2-3 days. We suggest longitudinal assessment of laboratory tests involving the RCV. This requires the application of standards of good laboratory practice. In this way the development of RFS can be observed promptly and in the initial phase can be easily corrected before developing symptoms.

References

[1] Boateng A, Sriram K, Meguid M, Crook M. Refeeding syndrome: treatment considerations based on collective analysis of literature case reports. *Nutrition* 2010; 26(2):156-67.

[2] National Institute for Health and Clinical Excellence. Clinical Guideline 32. Nutrition support in adults: oral nutrition support, enteral tube feeding and parenteral nutrition. 2006. Avliable at: *http://www.nice.org.uk/nicemedia/live/10978/29979/29979.pdf* Access on 10th July 2012.

[3] National Collaborating Centre for Acute Care, February 2006. Nutrition support in adults Oral nutrition support, enteral tube feeding and parenteral nutrition. National Collaborating Centre for Acute Care, London. Available from *http://www.rcseng.ac.uk* . Access on 10th July 2012.

[4] Mehanna HM, Moledina J, Travis J. Refeeding syndrome: What it is, and how to prevent and treat it. *BMJ* 2008;336:1495–98.

[5] Machado JD, Suen VM, Chueire FB, Marchini JF, Marchini JS. Refeeding syndrome, an undiagnosed and forgotten potentially fatal condition. [Electronic version]. BMJ Case Rep. 2009; doi: 10.1136/bcr.07.2008.0521. Available at: *http://www.ncbi.nlm.nih.gov/pmc/articles/PMC3028379/?tool =pubmed*. Accessed on July 17th 2012.

[6] Stanga Z, Brunner A, Leuenberger M, Grimble RF, Shenkin A, Allison SP, Lobo DN. Nutrition in clinical practice - the refeeding syndrome: illustrative cases and guidelines for prevention and treatment. *Eur J Clin Nutr* 2008;62: 687–94.

[7] Khan LUR, Ahmed J, Khan S, MacFie J. Refeeding Syndrome: A Literature Review. [Electronic version]. Gastroenterol Res Pract 2011. doi:10.1155/2011/410971. Available at: *http://www.ncbi.nlm.nih.gov /pmc/articles/PMC2945646/*. Accessed on July 17th 2012.

[8] Camp MA, Allon M. Severe hypophosphatemia in hospitalised patients. *Mineral & Electrolyte Metabolism* 1990;16:365-8.

[9] Afzal NA, Addai S, Fagbemi A, Murch S, Thomson M, Heuschel R. Refeeding syndrome with enteral nutrition in children:a case report, literature review and clinical guidelines. *Clin Nutr* 2002; 21(6): 515–20.

[10] Gonzalez AG, Fajardo-Rodriguez A, Gonzalez-Figueroa E. The incidence of the refeeding syndrome in cancer patients who receive artificial nutritional treatment (English abstract). *Nutr Hosp.* 1996;11:98.

[11] Berg JM, Tymoczko JL, Stryer L. *Biochemistry.* 5th edition. New York: W H Freeman; 2002.

[12] Dickerson RN. Guidelines for the Intravenous Management of Hypophosphatemia, Hypomagnesemia, Hypokalemia, and Hypocalcemia. *Hosp Pharm* 2001;36(11):1201–8.

[13] Levi M, Popovtzer M. Disorders of Phosphate Balance. In: Schrier RW, Berl T, Bonventre JV, eds. *Atlas of Diseases of the Kidney* (1), Current Medicine, Philadelphia PA; 1999. P.7.1–7.14

[14] Mehanna H, Nankivell PC, Moledina J, Travis J. Refeeding syndrome – awareness, prevention and managemen. [Electronic version]. Head Neck Oncol 2009; 1: 4. doi:10.1186/1758-3284-1-4 . Available at: *http://www.headandneckoncology.org/content/1/1/4*. Accessed Mart 18, 2012.

[15] Gennari FJ. Hypokalemia. *N Engl J Med.* 1998;339:451–8.

[16] Dacey MJ. Hypomagnesemic disorders.*Crit Care Clin.* 2001;17:155–73.

[17] Carlstedt F, Lind L. Hypocalcemic syndromes. *Crit Care Clin* 2001;17:139–53.

[18] Fattal-Valevski A. Thiamine (Vitamin B1). [Electronic version]. J Evid Based Complementary Altern Med 2011;16: 12-20. doi: 10.1177/1533210110392941. Available at: *http://chp.sagepub.com /content/16/1/12*. Accessed on July 17th 2012.

[19] Ricós C, Perich C, Minchinela J, Alvarez V, Simon M, Biosca C, et al. Application of biological variation - a review. *Biochem Med* 2009;19:250-9.

[20] Fraser CG. The utility of population-based reference values. In: *Biological Variation: From Principles to Practice.* Washington: AACC Press; 2001; 91-117.

[21] Ricos C, Alvarez V, Cava F, Garcia-Lario JV, Hernandez A, Jimenez CV, at al. Minimum Specifications for Total Error, Imprecision, and Bias, derived from intra- and inter-individual biologic variation. The 2012 update. Avaliable at: *http://www.westgard.com/minimum-biodatabase1.htm*. Accessed on 30th June 2012.

[22] Ricós C, Cava F, García-Lario JV, Hernández A, Iglesias N, Jimenez CV, et al. The reference change value: a proposal to interpret laboratory reports in serial testing based on biological variation. *Scand J Clin Lab Invest* 2004;64:175-84.

[23] Fraser CG. Changes in serial result. In: *Biological Variation: From Principles to Practice.* Washington: AACC Press; 2001; 67-91.

[24] *WHO guidelines on drawing blood: best practices in phlebothomy.* Printed by the WHO Document Production Servis, Geneva, Switzerland, 2010. Avaliable at:*http://whqlibdoc.who.int/publications /2010/9789241 599221_ eng.pdf.* Accessed on July 16th 2012.

[25] Clinical and Laboratory Standards Institute (CLSI*): Procedures for the Collection of Diagnostic Blood Specimens by Venipuncture — Sixth Edition (H3-A6)* November 2007; Avaliable at: *http://www.clsi.org /source/orders/free/h3-a6.pdf. Accessed July 16th 2012.* Accessed on July 16th 2012.

[26] Akobeng AK, Thomas AG. Refeeding syndrome following exclusive enteral nutritional treatment in Crohn disease. *J Pediatr Gastroenterol Nutr* 2010;51(3): 364-6.

[27] Agarwal J; Poddar U; Yachha SK; Srivastava A Refeeding syndrome in children in developing countries who have celiac disease. *J Pediatr Gastroenterol Nutr* 2012;54(4):521-4.

[28] Kolaček S. Treatment methods goals in pediatrics malnutrition. Ann Nestle 2009;67:85-93. Kolaček S. Treatment methods goals in pediatrics malnutrition. *Ann Nestle* 2009;67:85-93.

[29] Puntis JWL. Malnutrition in developed countries. *Ann Nestle* 2009;67:65-72.

[30] Mehanna HM, Moledina J,Travis J. Refeeding syndrome: What it is, and how to prevent and treat it. *BMJ* 2008;336(7659):1495–98.

[31] Cape Town Metrople Paediatric Interesting Group: *Refeedin syndrome: Guidelines.* Cape Town Metrople Paediatric Interesting Group. 2009.

[32] Stepan Giljevic J, Lenicek Krleza J, Jakovljevic G, Bonevski A, Jadrijevic Cvrlje F. Nutritional status in children with high-risk brain tumor: Diagnostic and therapeutic possibilities. *Pediatr Blood Cancer,* (Abstract) 44th Congress of the International Society of Paediatric Oncology (SIOP) 2012.

[33] Lenicek Krleza J, Misak Z, Jadresin O, Skaric I. Refeeding syndrome in children with different clinical aetiology. *European journal of clinical nutrition* 2013;67(8):883-6.

[34] Martinez MJ, Matrinez MA, Montero M, Campelo E, Castro I, Inaraja MT. Hypophosphatemia in postoperative patients on total parenteral nutrition: influence of nutritional support teams. *Nutr Hosp* 2006;21:657-60.

[35] Marik PE,Bedigan MK.Refeeding hypophosphataemia in an intensive care unit: a prospective study. *Arch Surg* 1996;131:1043-7.

[36] Santana e Meneses JF, Leite HP, de Carvalho WB, Lopes E. Hypophosphatemia in critically ill children: prevalence and associated risk factors.*Pediatr Crit Care Med* 2009;10:234-8.

[37] Ruiz Magro P, Aparicio Lopez C, Lopez-Herce Cid J, Martinez Campos M, Sancho Perez L. Metabolic changes in critically ill children. *An Esp Pediatr* 1999;51:143-8.

[38] Willis TS, Boswell R. Refeeding syndrome in a severely malnourished Child. *Laboratory Medicine* 2004:35(9):548-52.

[39] Klein S, Jeejeebhoy KN. The malnourished patient: Nutritional assessment and management. In: Feldman M, Friedman LS, Sleisenger MH, eds. Sleisenger & Fordtran's *Gastrointestinal and Liver Disease.* 7th ed. Philadelphia: WB Saunders Co; 2002. pp. 265–85.

[40] Botrán Prieto M, López-Herce CJ. Malnutrition in the Critically Ill Child: The Importance of Enteral Nutrition. *Int J Environ Res Public Health* 2011, 8:4353-66.

[41] Antachopoulos A, Margeli A, Giannaki M, Bakoula C, Liakopoulou T, Papassotiriou I. Transient hyopophosphataemia associated with acute infectious disease in paediatric patients. *Scand J Infect Dis* 2002; 34:836–39.

[42] Husby S, Koletzko S, Korponay-Szabo IR, Mearin ML, Phillips A, Shamir R at al. Coeliac Disease Diagnosis, on behalf of the ESPGHAN Gastroenterology Committee. European Society for Pediatric Gastroenterology, Hepatology, and Nutrition.Guidelines for the Diagnosis of Coeliac Disease. *J Pediatr Gastroenterol Nutr* 2012,54:136-60.

[43] Guideline for the Diagnosis and Treatment of Celiac Disease in Children: Recommendations of the North American Society for Pediatric Gastroenterology, Hepatology and Nutrition. J Pediatr Gastroenterol Nutr 2005. Available at: *http://www.naspghan.org/user-assets/Documents/pdf/PositionPapers/celiac_guideline_2004_jpgn.pdf,* Accessed on 10th July 2012.

[44] Donaldson MR, Firth SD, Wimpee H, Leiferman KM, ZoneJJ, Horsley W, at al. Correlation of duodenal histology with tissue transglutaminase

and endomysial antibody levels in pediatric celiac disease. *Clin Gastroenterol Hepatol* 2007;5:567-73.

[45] Barker CC, Mitton C, Jevon G, Mock T. Can tissue transglutaminase antibody titers replace small-bowel biopsy to diagnose celiac disease in select pediatric populations? *Pediatrics* 2005;115:1341-46.

[46] Vivas S, Ruiz de Morales JG, Riestra S, Arias L, Fuentes D, Alvarez N, at al. Duodenal biopsy may be avoided when high transglutaminase antibody titers are present. *World J Gastroenterol* 2009;15:4775-80.

[47] Lenicek Krleza J. Refeedin syndrome: What does it realy mean? In: *New Trends in Classification, Monitoring and Management of Gastrointestinal Diseases.* Editors: Topic E, Watson I, Homsak E, Lenicek Krleza J. Medicnska naklada, Zagreb, 2012.

Index

A

B

C

D

E

F

G

H

I

J

K

L

M

N

O

P

Q

R

S

T

U

V

W

X

Y

Z